Renal Diet Cookbook

200+ kidney friendly recipes to help you stay Healthy

By

Elizabeth Lopez

Contents

I would like to thank you for buying my book. I highly appreciate that. By the way, I would like to invite you to my Facebook group, where great gifts and news are waiting for you. Go get yours!

https://www.facebook.com/groups/elizabethlopezgroup

Introduction

The kidneys' main feature is to get rid of the body's toxins and excess fluid. They also (i) regulate minerals in the body, including salt & potassium, (ii) regulate fluids of the body, and (iii) produce hormones that influence other organs to function. Around a million filtering units or nephrons makeup one of the kidneys. A filter named the glomerulus & a tubule make a nephron. The nephrons function in a two-step process: the blood is drained by the glomerulus, & the tubule delivers the necessary materials to the blood and eliminates waste.

A long-term illness during which the kidneys do not work to their full capacity is chronic kidney disease. There is a very strong risk that you will eventually lose kidney function if you have chronic kidney disease (CKD). This illness sometimes gets worse slowly over time, rather than the disease making any immediate or dramatic changes. For chronic kidney disease, there is currently no proven treatment, but there are habits and activities which can reduce the progression of renal failure, including lifestyle behaviors. If you already suffer from diabetes, heart disease, high blood pressure, or have a history of kidney failure, you are at risk for kidney disease. If you already have risk factors, get screened for kidney failure and focus on making good eating habits, getting more active, striving for a healthy weight, and controlling health problems that cause kidney damage, and maintain your kidneys. Poor dietary patterns, smoking, and obesity are related to inclined risk danger kidney issues, as indicated by a new study published in the American Journal of Kidney Disease owned by National Kidney Foundation's Research conducted by Alex Chang, MD, who is the MS of Johns Hopkins University revealed that individuals with normal kidney work whose diet quality was poor that is high in red & processed meats, sugar drinks & sodium, & also low in natural food items such as vegetables, nuts, grains & low-fat dairy were more likely to get kidney disease.

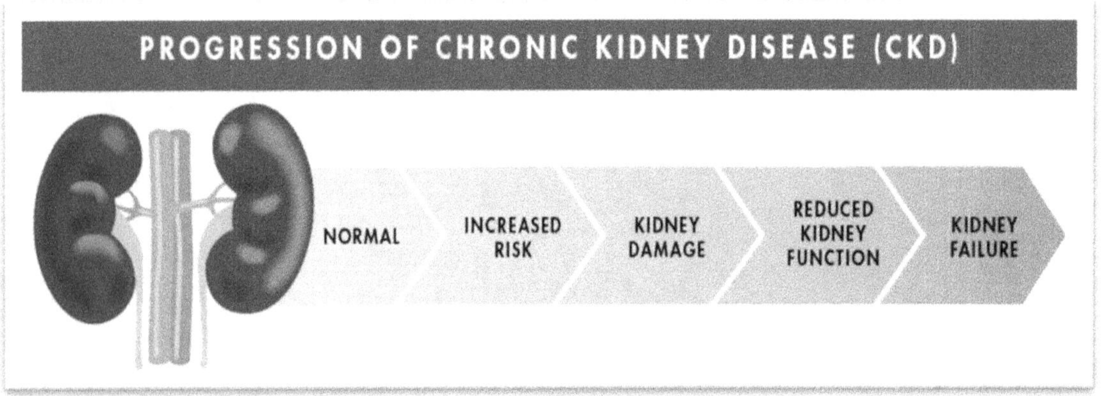

In chronic kidney disease (CKD) outcomes, diet plays a critical role. In persons with end-stage renal disease (ESRD), protein-energy wasting & inflammation are among the major risk factors for death. In those people with mild - to - moderate levels of kidney failure, the diet may be directly or indirectly linked scientifically with key components of CKD treatment, including blood pressure regulation and dyslipidemia management, diabetes. Diet influences a wide range of variables related to CKD treatment; it is important for the management of patients with CKD to consider the quality and quantity of foods that a person consumes. Several recent scientific journals have concentrated on the influence of diet on CKD outcomes. The main factor driving the development of obesity with major implications for long-term kidney function is excess calorie consumption. Maintaining a safe weight is part of the existing dietary recommendations for improving CKD outcomes, partially by decreased calorie consumption. For people with mild to serious kidney disease who are not on dialysis to delay the development of CKD, restriction of animal protein consumption is often advised. The consumption of micronutrients, such as sodium and phosphorus, has also been reported as a major contributor to the outcomes of CKD. Large clinical studies have shown that excess consumption of salt is linked to adverse clinical outcomes such as hypertension, volume overload & incidents of coronary disease. Excessive intake of phosphorus has long been involved in kidney disease pathogenesis. In animals with experimentally induced kidney disease, lower phosphorus consumption decreased the progression of kidney disease and increased longevity. This has backed recent guidelines to reduce the consumption of phosphorus in people with CKD,29, but it is unknown the target dose and best way to reach this level.

A kidney-friendly or renal diet is a healthy diet that serves to protect kidneys against damage. It is essential to ensure that one must get the correct levels of nutrients, calories, vitamins, and minerals. There may be few restrictions on what one should consume when experiencing the early stages of CKD. But one must be much more cautious about what is going in the bloodstream when the condition grows stronger.

 The doctor can recommend picking easy foods for the kidneys. Perhaps they would recommend to:

Reduced sodium intake: In many foods, sodium is present naturally. The most popular one is table salt. The blood pressure is impaired by sodium. It also allows the water throughout the body to be balanced. Safe kidneys hold normal amounts of sodium. Although in the case of CKD, the body accumulates additional sodium & fluids. It can exacerbate various conditions of the heart and lungs, such as swelling of knees, elevated blood pressure, fluid buildup, and shortness of breath. In a regular diet, one must strive for fewer than 2 grams of sodium.

To cut the salt in your diet, follow these basic steps:

- Stop table salt and seasonings with excessive sodium levels.

- Cook at home — many fast foods have a high sodium content.

- Instead of salt, try fresh herbs.

- Where necessary, abstain from processed goods. They seem to be sodium-rich.

- When shopping, read all labeling, and select low-sodium items.

- Before eating, wash canned foods with water.

To keep your bones safe and solid, you need minerals such as calcium and phosphorus. They extract the phosphorus you do not use to keep kidneys healthy. But the phosphorus levels might get too high in CKD. It creates a risk of heart failure. Furthermore, the levels of calcium start to decline. The body may pull everything from the bones to cover allowances for it. It will weaken them and make them easier to crack. The doctor may recommend getting amounts of not more than 1,000 milligrams (mg) of phosphorus mineral per day in late-stage CKD. It can be achieved by:

- Having chosen foods with low phosphorus levels

- Consuming additional new vegetables and fruit

- Selecting cereals including corn and rice

- Light-colored drinking sodas

- Trying to cut back on beef, seafood, and poultry.

- Restriction of dairy foods

Foods rich in calcium happen to be high in phosphorus as well. The doctor may suggest cutting back on foods high in calcium. Dairy foods with lower phosphorus content include:

- Brie / Swiss cheese

- Standard or low-fat cheese for milk/sour cream

- Sherbet

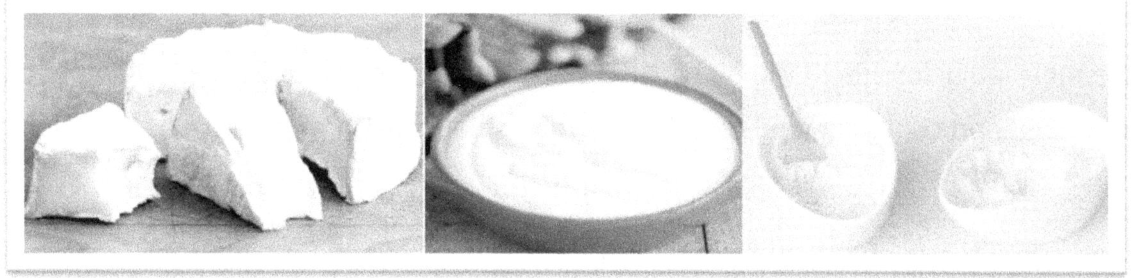

Reduce the consumption of potassium. It helps to improve the function of muscles and nerves. Yet, the body cannot flush all the excess potassium in CKD. It can lead to severe cardiac attacks when. Doctors might propose to seek low-potassium foods, including:

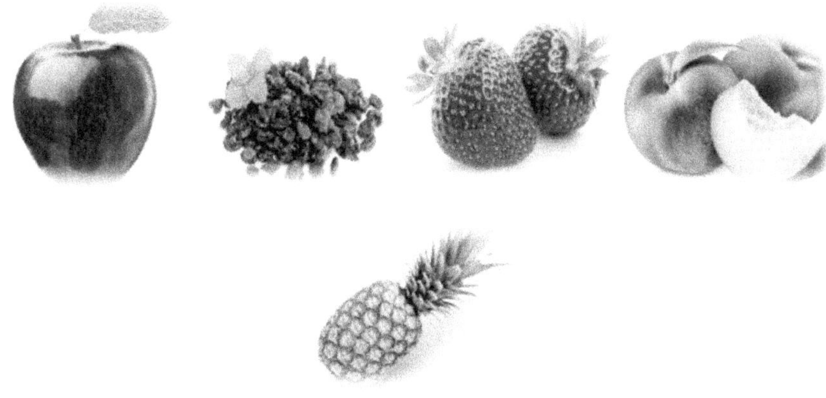

- Apples or apple juice

- Cranberries or juice of cranberries

- Strawberry, blueberry, raspberry

- Peaches

- Plums

- Pineapples

- Cabbage

- Beans (green or wax)

- Boiled cauliflower

- Asparagus

- Cucumber

- Celery

One must make more adjustments to the diet if CKD becomes worse. It may mean cutting back on high-protein foods, particularly animal protein. It involves items such as beef, fish, including dairy.

This book will provide a range of kidney-friendly recipes that will help you maintain sodium, phosphorus, and potassium levels in the body. The recipes include many options for breakfast, lunch, and dinner. It also provides easy to make and delicious recipes for snacks, salads, desserts, and beverages. Preparation time, calorie intake, and difficulty levels of the recipes are also provided to support you and your family.

Chapter 1: Kidney friendly Renal Diet Breakfast Recipes

1. Egg Muffin Cups

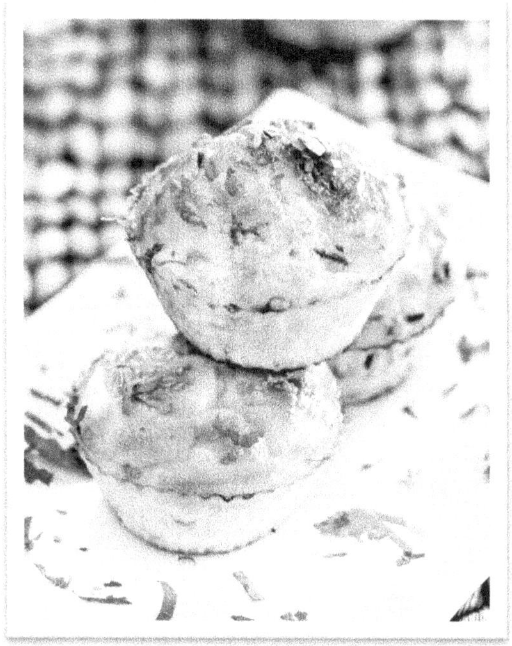

Calories: 59cal |Total time: 40min| Servings: 12 | Difficulty: Easy

Ingredients

- Vegetables 1 cup, use them as nicely diced small or shredded (you can use squash, carrot and yellow or red pepper)

- Oil, 1 Teaspoon

- Eggs, 8

- fresh herbs, 1 Tablespoon (basil and parsley can be used)

- Green and white, 3 whole stalks, must be thinly sliced use green onions or scallions

- Mayo, 2 Teaspoon

- Small slices of brie, (optional)

- Lemon zest as per taste (~1 Teaspoon)

Instruction

1. Sautee vegetables in the oil until they are softened. Put them aside to cool. Whisk eggs

and mayonnaise together in a cup. Add the spices and the green onions.

2. Transfer roasted vegetables. Place them in 12 separate muffin tins.

3. Now top with a tiny slice of brie (optional). Silicon muffin tin is better, so muffins will quickly pop out of them. You might make it in a 9×9 dish for a casserole meal.

4. Bake it around 350 F for around 20-25 minutes or until each muffin's core is properly set. Apply the lemon zest to the top of every muffin.

5. Enjoy!

2. Dilly Scrambled Eggs

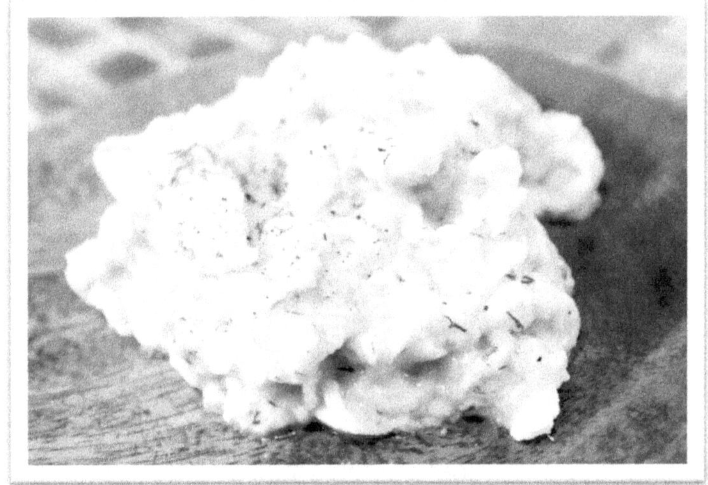

|Calories: 194 |Total time: 10min | Servings: 2 | Difficulty: Easy

Ingredients

- Large eggs, 2

- Black pepper, 1/8 teaspoon

- Dried dill weed, 1 teaspoon

- Crumbled goat cheese, 1 tablespoon

Instruction

1. Start by beating the eggs in a medium bowl; put in a non-stick pan over medium heat.

2. Add the black pepper after some time, and then add dill to the egg.

3. Cook until the eggs have scrambled.

4. Cover with goat cheese right before serving.

5. Enjoy.

3. Breakfast Bagel

|Calories: 134 |Total time: 10min| Servings: 2 | Difficulty: Easy

Ingredients

- 2-ounce size bagel 1,

- Cream cheese, 2 tablespoons

- 1/4-inch-thick slices of 2 tomatoes,

- Slices of 2 red onion

- Lemon-pepper seasoning (low-sodium) 1 teaspoon

Instruction

1. Slice the bagel and toast it until you see a nice golden color.

2. Layer the cream cheese over half of each bagel.

3. Place the onions and tomato (sliced) on top of the bagel, finally sprinkle the lemon pepper as seasoning.

4. Serve.

4. Apple Oatmeal Custard

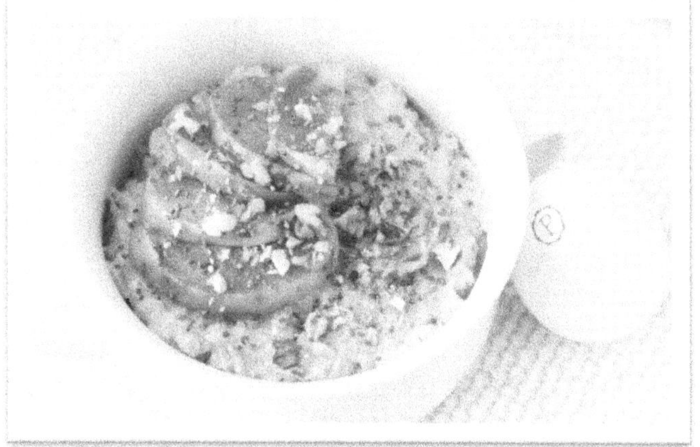

|Calories:248 |Total time: 6min | Servings: 1| Difficulty: Easy

Ingredients

- Oatmeal (quick cooking), 1/3 cup

- Large, egg 1

- Almond milk, 1/2 cup

- Cinnamon, 1/4 teaspoon

- A medium-size apple 1/2

Instruction

1. Start by cutting the apple in half, finely cut in slices.

2. In a big bowl, mix peas, egg, and almond milk. Then stir with fork. Now add cinnamon and sliced apple to the mixture.

3. Stir again before the combination is fully blended.

4. Cook at high temperature in a microwave for around 2 minutes. When It is felt Fluff with a fork, it has almost done. You may Cook for another 30 to 60 seconds, if necessary.

5. Stir in a little extra milk or water in case you feel the cereal is thinner.

5. Egg Scramble Coffee Cup

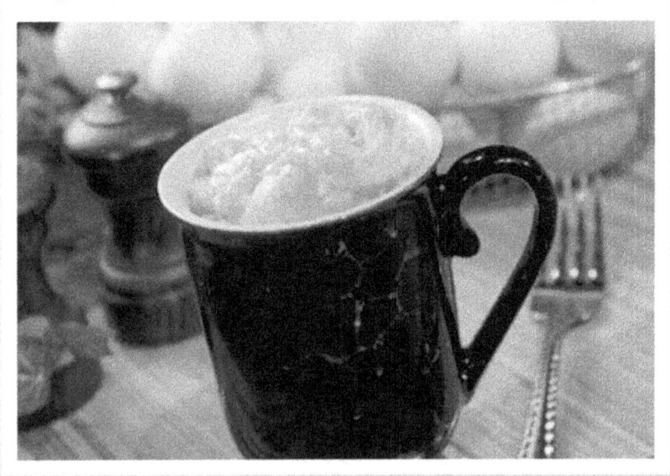

|Calories:117 | Total time: 7min | Servings: 1 | Difficulty: Easy

Ingredients

- Large egg, 1

* Egg whites of 2 large eggs

* 1% low-fat milk, 2 tablespoons

* Black pepper, 1/8 teaspoon

Instruction

1. Use any cooking spray to spray a 12-ounce cup using this spray. In the mug, mix the sugar, egg, and egg whites, then beat until mixed.

2. Put a coffee cup into the microwave and cook it for 45 seconds; remove and mix well. Microwave again for 30-45 seconds before the eggs are almost ready.

3. Sprinkle with the pepper and taste it.

4. You may add 1/4 cup of sliced onion or bell pepper and mushrooms for extra flavor.

6. French Toast Microwave Egg White

|Calories:200 |Total time: 10min | Servings: 1 | Difficulty: Easy

Ingredients

* 1 slice of bread

* Unsalted butter 1 teaspoon, softened

* Egg whites, 1/2 cup

* Sugar-free syrup, 2 tablespoons

Instruction

1. Pour butter on bread or muffin. Split into cubes.

2. Use a microwave-safe dish and put buttered bread cubes inside.

3. Top with egg whites over the bread to coat them.

4. Sprinkle the sugar on top of that.

5. Microwave for about 1 minute; press up the white egg edges so that the uncooked egg spread on the dish's ground.

6. Microwave for another 1 minute or until the egg is fully set.

7. Kidney friendly breakfast Omelet

|Calories:117 | Total time:15min | Servings: 2 | Difficulty: Easy

Ingredients

- Eggs, 2

- Non-dairy creamer, 2 tablespoons

- Diced bell peppers and onions,2

- Fresh ground pepper as per taste

- Paprika according to taste

- Shredded cheddar cheese, 1 tablespoon

Instruction

1. Prepare a shallow non-stick skillet and spray on it a non-stick spray.

2. Beat the eggs, the spices and the non-dairy creamer using a small cup until frothy.

3. In the pan, set heat to low, and Sautee the pepper and onion until cooked through. Pour the egg mixture over the onions and the pepper.

4. Tilt the egg mixture to cook uniformly.

5. Allow setting halfway right before the cheese is sprinkled. When the omelet has been settled, fold in half, then serve with toast slice.

8. Breakfast French Toast

|Calories:125 | Total time: 15min| Servings:1 | Difficulty: Easy

Ingredients

- White bread, 2 slices

- Egg whites of 2 eggs

- Non-dairy creamer, 1 tablespoon

- Cinnamon, 1 small piece

- Pure maple syrup, 1 tablespoon

- Fresh berries, ¼ cup

Instruction

1. Spray any non-sticky spray to prepare a non-stick skillet and heat on low flame.

2. Start beating the egg whites slowly with some cinnamon and the creamer while the pan is being heated.

3. Place the piece of bread in the egg mixture and cover both sides with the mixture. Put the coated bread in the skillet, now cook the bread until the golden-brown color is achieved.

4. Finally, Drizzle with the maple syrup and garnish with new berries like blueberries or strawberries.

9. Breakfast Sausage patties

|Calories:173| Total time: 35min | Servings: 16 |Difficulty: Medium

Ingredients

- Finely chopped onion, 1⁄2 cup

- Olive oil, 2 tablespoons

- Dried sage, 2 teaspoons

- Fresh ground black pepper, 1 teaspoon

- White sugar or brown sugar, 1 tablespoon

- Red pepper flakes crushed, 1⁄8 teaspoon

- Ground cloves, 1 pinch

- Finely chopped fresh thyme1 teaspoon,

- Egg yolk, 1 large egg

- Lean meat, 2-lbs

Instruction

1. Cook the onion using olive oil for about 8-10 minutes over relatively low heat.

2. Stir regularly until the onion begins to soften and get brown.

3. Now Cool them for about 10 minutes.

4. In a small cup, mix red and black pepper, sage, sugar, cloves, and thyme.

5. Put the egg yolk on meat with some onion in a wide tub, then add all the mixed spices. Then Mix everything well and shape into 16 patties, two ounces each.

6. Finally, Cook the patties in a wide skillet over medium heat for about 5 minutes to cook both sides or till the internal temperature exceeds 160 degrees.

10. Stuffed Breakfast Biscuits

|Calories: 330 | Total time: 25min | Servings: 1 | Difficulty: Medium

Ingredients

- Flour, 2 cups

- Sugar (or honey), 1 tablespoon

- Baking soda, ½ teaspoon

- Lemon juice, 1 tablespoon

- Unsalted butter, 8 tablespoons softened

- Milk, ¾ cup

Filling:

- Eggs, 4

- Bacon, (1¼ chopped) reduced sodium 8 ounces

- Cheddar cheese, 1 cup

- Thinly sliced scallions, ¼ cup

Instruction

Preheat your oven to 425° F.

Prepare the filling:

1. Scrambled eggs are somewhat undercooked.

2. Heat the bacon until it is crispy.

3. Mix with the four components and put them aside.

Prepare the dough:

1. In a wide bowl, mix all the dry ingredients.

2. Break the non-salted butter using a fork or pastry knife until it becomes pea-size or smaller.

3. Create a well in the middle of the mixture and knead with the lemon juice and the milk.

4. Prepare the muffin tins with lining or gently grease with flour on the bottom and the sides.

5. Scoop ¼ cup of the mixture into muffin tins.

6. Finally, bake for about 10-12 minutes at 425°F or till it becomes golden brown.

11. Turkey Breakfast Burritos

|Calories:407 | Total time: 15min | Servings: 8 | Difficulty: Easy

Ingredients

- Ground turkey, 1-pound or use leftover turkey meatloaf 1-pound, small cubed

- Flour burrito shells, 8 6-inch

- Canola oil, ¼ cup

- Scrambled beaten eggs, 8

- Diced onions, ¼ cup

- Fresh bell peppers, ¼ cup (yellow, red, or green) diced

- Seeded jalapeno peppers, 2 tablespoons

- Chopped fresh scallions, 2 tablespoons

- Chopped fresh cilantro, 2 tablespoons

- Chili powder, ½ teaspoon

- Smoked paprika, ½ teaspoon

- Shredded cheddar cheese and Monterey jack 1 cup

Instruction

1. sauté meatloaf and onions with tomatoes; after some time, add scallions and cilantro in it and cook until translucent. Mix in the spices and decrease the heat.

2. Set heat to medium and put another large saucepan on flame, then add the oil and scrambled eggs.

3. Put the same quantity of vegetables and meatloaf mixture, eggs, and cheese, and finally, fold them and serve in burrito shells.

12. Breakfast Blueberry Muffins

|Calories:275 | Total time: 45min | Servings:12muffin |Difficulty: Medium

Ingredients

- Unsalted butter, ½ cup

- Cups sugar, 1 ¼

- Eggs, 2

- 1% milk, 2 cups

- All-purpose flour, 2 cups

- Baking powder, 2 teaspoons

- Salt, ½ teaspoon

- Fresh blueberries, 2 ½ cups

- Sugar (for topping), 2 teaspoons

Instruction

1. Use a low-speed processor, blend the margarine and sugar until smooth and fluffy.

2. Add the eggs one by one (only one at a time) and stir until completely mixed).

3. Sift the dry ingredients, then add the milk one after another.

4. Mash 1/2 cup of blueberries and again stir by hand. Then add all the remaining blueberries and mix by hand.

5. Spray the muffin cups and the top of the vegetable oil tray. Put the muffins in the tin.

6. Pile the muffin mixture higher in - the cup of muffin. Sprinkle the sugar over the muffin layer.

7. Bake about 25–30 min at 375°F. Cool in the pan for at least 25 minutes before extracting.

13. Moon Pie Stuffing with Chocolate Pancakes

|Calories:194 | Total time: 1hour | Servings: 12 | Difficulty: Medium

Ingredients

Moon Pie Stuffing:

- Cocoa powder unsweetened, 1 tablespoon

- Heavy cream, ¼ cup

- Cream cheese softened, ½ cup

- Marshmallow cream, ½ cup

Chocolate Pancakes:

- Flour, 1 cup

- Sugar, 3 tablespoons

- Cocoa powder unsweetened, 3 tablespoons

- Baking soda, ½ teaspoon

- Lemon juice, 1 tablespoon

- Egg, 1

- 2% milk, 1 cup

- Canola oil, 2 tablespoons

- Vanilla extract, 2 teaspoons

- Body fortress whey protein powder, 2/3 cup (vanilla)

Instruction

1. Beat cocoa powder and heavy cream until rigid peaks have developed.

2. Whip in cream cheese with marshmallow cream, then add whey protein powder and mix well for around a minute or until properly mixed, but do not overbeat. Cover and put aside in the

refrigerator.

Pancakes:

3. In a wide cup, mix all the dry form ingredients and set aside.

4. Mix all the moist ingredients in a medium dish.

5. Gradually put dry ingredients in a mixture of wet ingredients when wet, but do not over-mix.

6. Cook the pancakes using a finely oiled griddle over medium heat, around 375°F.

7. Use around 1/8 of the batter's cup to produce 4-inch pancakes, rotating as the bubble begins to pop up.

---

14. Fluffy Buttermilk Pancakes

|Calories: 217 | Total time: 20min | Servings: 9 | Difficulty: Easy

Ingredients

- All-purpose flour, 2 cups

- Cream of tartar, 1 teaspoon

- Baking soda, 1½ teaspoons

- Sugar, 2 tablespoons

- Low-fat buttermilk, 2 cups

- Eggs, 2 large size

- Canola oil, ¼ cup and canola oil (for cooking), 1 tablespoon

Instruction

1. Buttermilk, with some oil and egg mixture, then use a fork or a spoon to combine the dry ingredients mix well or until they are fully wet.

2. Use one tablespoon of canola oil for greasing. Add a Scoop of pancake mixture into the skillet using 1/3 of a measuring cup. Each pancake is expected to stretch to around 4 inches across.

3. Leave about 2-inch space between the pancakes to flip them quickly. Flip the pancakes with a spatula continue this process until the bubbles are completely gone from the top of

the pancake. Make the other side brown or until the middle is no longer wet.

4. Shift to serve the cup.

5. You may think about serving with new berries or eggs for a better twist.

6. Tip: Freeze the remaining buttermilk pancakes in the refrigerator, which may be reheated for a simple breakfast.

15. Cheesesteak Quiche

|Calories: 527 | Total time: 20min | Servings: 6 | Difficulty: Easy

Ingredients

- Sirloin steak meat shaved, ½ pound coarsely chopped

- Diced onions, 1 cup

- Canola oil, 2 tablespoons

- Pepper jack cheese, ½ cup, shredded

- 5 eggs, beaten

- Cream, 1 cup

- Prepared piecrust*1" x 9" deep par-cooked

- Ground black pepper, ½ teaspoon

Instruction

1. Chop shaved sirloin into pieces.

2. In a Sautee pan, Sautee the sliced steak with onions and oil until the beef is browned. Put aside to cool for ten minutes. Fold the cheese, then let it settle.

3. In a wide cup, beat the eggs with cream and the black pepper until well combined.

4. Place the cheese mixture with steak on the base of par-cooked piecrust, now spill the egg mixture over it and bake at 350° F for about 30 minutes.

5. Cover the cheesesteak quiche with foil and turn the oven off. Let the quiche be set for ten minutes, then serve.

16. Spicy Tofu Scrambler

|Calories:213 | Total time: 35min| Servings:2 | Difficulty: Easy

Ingredients

- Olive oil, 1 teaspoon

- Chopped red bell pepper, ¼ cup

- Chopped green bell pepper, ¼ cup

- Firm tofu, 1 cup (<10% calcium)

- Onion powder, 1 teaspoon

- Garlic powder, ¼ teaspoon

- Garlic, minced, 1 clove

- Turmeric, ⅛ teaspoon

Instruction

1. Use a medium-sized non-stick pan to sauté the garlic and the two bell peppers using some olive oil.

2. Rinse and well drain the tofu and cook it in a skillet.

3. Add all the ingredients to the skillet.

4. Stir and cook for few minutes on medium heat or until the tofu becomes golden brown. It will take around 20 minutes. Meanwhile, water is going to evaporate.

5. Serve the scrambler tofu wet.

17. Breakfast Cups Southwest Baked Egg

|Calories:109 | Total time: 25min | Servings: 12 | Difficulty: Medium

Ingredients

- Cooked rice, 3 cups

- Cheddar cheese, 4 ounces shredded

- Green chilies, diced 4 ounces

- Pimentos, 2 ounces drained and diced

- Skim milk, ½ cup

- 2 eggs, beaten

- Ground cumin, ½ teaspoon

- Black pepper, ½ teaspoon

- Some non-stick cooking sprays

Instruction

1. In a large-size bowl, combine the rice and 2 ounces of cheese with some chilies, onions, cumin cream, eggs, and pepper.

2. Spray the muffin cup with some amount of non-stick cooking spray.

3. Spread the mixture uniformly into 12 cups of muffin. Sprinkle the remaining 2 oz of melted cheese on top of every cup.

4. Bake at 400-degrees for about 15 minutes or until ready.

18. Maple Pancakes

|Calories:178 | Total time: 35min | Servings:5 | Difficulty: Easy

Ingredients

- All-purpose flour, 1 cup

- Granulated sugar, 1 tablespoon

- Baking powder, 2 teaspoons

- Salt, 1/8 teaspoon

- Egg whites of 2 large eggs

- 1% low-fat milk, 1 cup

- Canola oil, 2 tablespoons

- Maple extract, 1 tablespoon

Instruction

1. Mix rice, starch, bakery powder and salt together in a medium dish. In the middle of the dry ingredient's mixture, make a well.

2. Mix egg whites, sugar, olive oil and maple extract in a wide cup.

3. Add the egg blend to the dry blend at once. Remove before damp (batter may be lumpy).

4. Place 4" pancakes over a hot and slightly greased griddle. You may use a heavy skillet, too and use it for around 1/4 cup batter.

5. Cook about 2 min on each side, use medium heat for cooking, cook till the pancakes are golden.

6. Flip the breadcrumbs when it shows a slightly dry bubbling top. Turn only once and stop pushing with the spatula to retain pancakes lighter and fluffy.

19. Heavenly Challah

|Calories:144 | Total time: 2hour | Servings: 15| Difficulty: Medium

Ingredients

- All-purpose flour, 7 cups

- Dry baker's yeast, 2 tablespoons

- Sugar, 6 tablespoons

- Warm water, 2-1/2 cups

- Vegetable oil, 1/2 cup

- Salt, 2 teaspoons

- 1 large egg

Instruction

1. Through some large bowl, put together yeast and sugar with flour, water and oil to form a dough. Add some salt when a ball-shaped is formed. Place the prepared dough on a floured surface, knead it until it is smooth and non-sticky for 10 minutes.

2. Coat 1 to 2 tablespoons of oil in a bowl. Cover the bowl and put it in a warm place until the

dough is doubled (1 to 2 hours are required).

3. For a couple of minutes, knead the rose dough, then Cut the dough into Twelve sections and roll into a twined strand, around 10" or 12" long.

4. Three braids of rolling dough shape the challah together. Now repeat 4 challahs with other dough lines.

5. Place the baking sheet or bakery, cover the challenges, and let the dough rise again for about 40 minutes.

6. At 350 degrees F, preheated oven bakes for 30min. Brush with the beaten egg per challah. Bake until the challahs become golden brown for about 30 minutes. Finally, remove from the oven. It is ready to serve

20. Blueberry Squares

|Calories:247 |Total time: 1 hour | Servings: 16 | Difficulty: Easy

Ingredients

- Cups flour, 1 1/2

- Oats, 1 cup

- Cinnamon, 1 teaspoon

- Sugar, 1 cup

- Sticks melted butter, 3/4 cup or 1 1/2 (unsalted)

- Blueberries, 3 cups

- 1 lemon zest

- Cornstarch, 3 tablespoons

- Sugar, 3/4 cup

- Water, 1 cup

Instruction

1. Preheat the oven to 350 degrees.

2. In a medium dish, mix rice, peas, cinnamon, and sugar with butter until crumbling.

3. Press 1/2 flour with oat mixture into a 9-inch square plate.

4. Add the lemon zest with blueberries and cover the base of the plate.

5. Mix cornstarch and the sugar in a microwaveable dish, stir steadily in water, now heat it until boiling temperature is achieved.

6. Place the water, cornstarch, and sugar mixture over blueberries.

7. Top with the rest of the flour or oat mixture.

8. Cook for about 45 minutes or 1 hour, serve hot.

21. Lemon Apple Honey Smoothie

|Calories:170 | Total time: 5min | Servings: 4 | Difficulty: Easy

Ingredients

- Lemon juice, 1/4 cup

- Apple juice, 1/2 cup

- Peeled and cored apple, 1

- 1 banana

- Honey, 2-3 teaspoons

- Vanilla frozen yogurt, 1 cup

Instruction

1. Mix all ingredients in a blender, then blend on high speed until the mixture is smooth.

2. Pour in a big, chilled glass bottle.

22. Yeast Rolls

|Calories:148 | Total time: 45min | Servings: 20 | Difficulty: Easy

Ingredients

- Hot water, 1 cup

- Vegetable shortening, 6 tablespoons

- Sugar, ½ cup

- Yeast, 1 package

- Of warm water, 2 tablespoons

- 1 egg

- All-purpose flour, 3 ¾-4 cups

Instruction

1. Preheat the oven to 400 degrees F.

2. In a wide bowl, mix hot water with shortening and sugar. Put aside to cool in a safe place.

3. Dissolve the yeast in hot water.

4. Add the milk, yeast, and flour (only half of it) into the mixture, use a wide bowl and beat it well.

5. Mix the remaining flour using a spoon until it is simple to treat.

6. Place the dough in a bowl that is already greased and cover it with plastic wrap.

7. Allow to rest for 1 to 1 1/2 hours or till the dough becomes double in size.

8. Cut the sum into the required amount to shape the rolls.

9. Bake the rolls for about 12 minutes until it is completely cooked

23. Craisins with Baked Apples

|Calories:200 | Total time: 55min | Servings: 4 | Difficulty: Easy

Ingredients

- 2 apples

- Apple juice, 1 cup

- Brown sugar packed, ¼ cup

- Craisins, 2 tablespoons

- Few red cinnamons candy

Instruction

1. Preheat to 375 Fan ovens.

2. Clean the apples and put them aside.

3. Use a square pan (size 9" x 9" x 1 3⁄4"), add apple juice with brown sugar.

4. Place the apples in the pan.

5. Cover apple centers with craisins with some cinnamon candies.

6. Now Place the pan into the microwave. Spoon sometimes adds some juice over apples for glazing during baking to stop your apples from drying.

7. Bake for around 40 to 45 minutes or till the apples is crispy when punctured with a fork.

24. Pan Sausage

|Calories:96 |Total time: 10min | Servings: 6 | Difficulty: Easy

Ingredients

- Fresh lean ground meat (beef, chicken, or turkey), 1-pound

- Ground sage, 2 teaspoons

- Granulated sugar, 2 teaspoons

- Ground black pepper, 1 teaspoon

- Ground red pepper, ½ teaspoon

- Basil (optional), 1 teaspoon

- Cooking spray

Instruction

1. Demand the butcher for meat loins of your choice.

2. Mix all the ingredients well to render the sausage.

3. Measure 2 teaspoons of the meat mixture to render a patty.

4. Pan fry or broil it until cooked properly.

25. Mexican Egg & Tortilla Skillet Breakfast (Mega)

|Calories:297 | Total time: 10min | Servings:6 | Difficulty: Easy

Ingredients

- Eggs or eggbeaters, 8

- Green onions 2, make thin slices

- Chili powder, 1 teaspoon

- Low salt ketchup, 1/4 cup

- Butter, 2 tablespoons

- Unsalted tortilla chips 1 bag (6oz) *, broken up

Instruction

1. Beat the eggs until mixed.

2. Add the onion with chili powder and some ketchup. Beat again before it is well combined. Set it aside.

3. Melt some butter in a pan, then add tortilla chips and Sautee over medium heat until it is soft. Stir in the mixture of eggs and scramble till the ideal consistency is achieved. Serve hot.

* If you cannot locate unsalted tortilla chips, you may use flour tortillas and break them in fourths. Finally, Bake them until crisp at a temperature of 350°F.

26. Fresh Fruit Compote

| Calories:44| Total time: 15min | Servings: 8 | Difficulty: Easy

Ingredients

- Fresh or frozen strawberries, 1/2 cup

- Fresh or frozen blackberries, 1/2 cup

- Fresh or frozen blueberries,1/2 cup

- Pared, cut peaches, 1/2 cup

- Fresh or frozen red raspberries, 1/4 cup, sweetened but not thawed

- Fresh or canned, orange juice, 1/2 cup, unsweetened

- Apple, sliced into bite-size pieces 1

- Banana, 1 sliced into bite-size pieces

Instruction

1. Add orange juice in a big container.

2. Add all the ingredients and mix gently.

3. Allow resting at room temperature for 4 hours. For thawing, use frozen berries.

27. Mexican Sausage with Eggs and Burritos

|Calories:320k| Total time: 15min | Servings: 3 | Difficulty: Easy

Ingredients

- (Mexican sausage) chorizo, 3 ounces

- Beaten eggs, 3

- Flour tortillas, 3

Instruction

1. Fry chorizo in a medium sizes skillet until the color gets dark.

2. Add the eggs and cook them until done.

3. Fill the hot tortillas using the mixture and roll them up. Now fold the bottom edge while rolling to prevent the filling from spilling out.

4. The server right away.

28. Orange Flavored Coffee

|Calories:47k| Total time: 5min | Servings: 20 | Difficulty: Easy

Ingredients

- Instant coffee, 1/2 cup

- Sugar, 3/4 cup

- Coffee-mate powder 1 cup

- Dried orange peel, 1/2 teaspoon

Instruction

1. Blend all the listed ingredients using a high-speed blender until the powdered form is achieved.

2. Place 2 circular teaspoons of the coffee mixture in a cup with each serving; finally, add the Boiling water to it

29. Caramel Rolls

|Calories:137| Total time: 33min | Servings:24 | Difficulty: Medium-High

Ingredients

Sweet roll dough

- Flour, 2 c.
- Active dry yeast 1 pkg
- Skim milk, 1 c.
- Sugar, 1/3 c.
- Margarine, 3 Tablespoon.
- Salt, 1/4 Teaspoon
- Egg whites of 2
- Flour, 2 - 2 1/2 c.

Sauce

- Packed brown sugar, 1/2 c.
- Margarine, 3 tablespoons
- Light corn syrup 2 tablespoon
- Sugar, 1/3 c.
- Ground cinnamon, 1 teaspoon.
- Margarine melted, 1 tablespoon.

Instruction

1. Use a large bowl and add 2 cups of flour in it with yeast and set aside.

2. Mix milk, sugar, and margarine with some salt in a small size saucepan.

3. Heat and stir the mixture over low heat to melt margarine; once melted, add it to the flour blend.

4. Add whites of egg, now beat the eggs for 30 seconds with electrical beater, at medium speed, then beat for 50 seconds or more at full speed.

5. Use a spoon and add 2 – 2 1/2 cups of flour to it.

6. Knead the residual flour on a washed surface with some flour roughly spread for making a smooth dough. You will need moderately soft dough, which will be made in 3 to 5 minutes.

7. Shape the dough into a ball.

8. Spray cooking oil in a large non-stick coated bowl. Put the dough; turn it once.

9. Cover the dough with a cloth and let it rise by placing it in a warm area for about an hour; it should be twice the original size. Punch down dough with a toothpick, turn to a slightly blurred surface.

10. Split the dough into half.

11. Cover and leave 10 minutes to rest.

12. When the dough rises, mix brown sugar in a small-sized saucepan, add 3 Tablespoons. Margarine.

13. Add Maize syrup. Cook and mix the compound until the margarine is fully melted and mix. Divide dough between 2 9-inch panels

14. Spread across panes; set aside panels.

15. Use a small bowl and mix sugar with cinnamon together.

16. Roll half of the dough into a triangle measuring 12 x 8 inches.

17. Brush it with margarine previously melted; sprinkle a little bit of sugar and some cinnamon.

18. Roll up like a jelly roll look from 1 side of the rim. Pinch edges to seal together.

19. Roll cut the pieces into twelve bits. In the previously prepared panes, put cut sides down.

20. Repeat the same process with the other half leftover dough. Now Cover it with a clean dish

towel, then allow to restore about 30 minutes.

21. Preheat the oven at 375°F pinch any bubble with a greased toothpick on the surface.

22. Bake for 20 minutes in a 375 °F oven bakes until sounding hollow when lightly tapped.

23. Invert the rolls on the platters to be served.

30. Apple Cinnamon Maple Granola

|Calories:162| Total time: 2hour | Servings:2 | Difficulty: Easy

Ingredients

- Puffed rice cereal, 3 cups

- Old fashioned oats, 3 cups

- Apple chips baked, 3.4-ounce package

- Sweetened cranberries dried, 1/2 cup

- Ground cinnamon, 1-1/2 teaspoons

- Ground nutmeg, 1 teaspoon

- Coconut oil melted, 1/4 cup

- Maple syrup pure, 1/4 cup

- Vanilla extract, 1-1/2 teaspoons

- Apple sauce unsweetened, 1/2 cup

Instruction

1. Preheat your oven around 275 F. Line 2 wide sheets of parchment paper for baking.

2. In a wide bowl, mix the dried ingredients.

3. In a small cup, combine the wet ingredients.

4. Pour the wet ingredients into a bowl of dried ingredients. To coat the dry ingredients, blend them well.

5. Using 2 baking sheets, break the mixture into half.

6. Bake for 60 to 65 minutes, adjusting the pan's position (moving the pan to the lower rack

from the top rack) halfway through the baking process.

---

31. Apple Onion Omelet

|Calories:284| Total time: 20min | Servings: 2 | Difficulty: Easy

Ingredients

- Eggs, 3 larges

- Low-fat milk (1%), 1/4 cup

- Water, 1 tablespoon

- Black pepper, 1/8 teaspoon

- Butter, 1 tablespoon

- Sweet onion, 3/4 cup

- Apple, 1 large

- 2 tablespoons cheddar cheese shredded

Instruction

1. Preheat the oven to around 400 degrees F.

2. Peel the apple make thin slices of apple and the onion.

3. Beat the eggs using a small bowl with milk, some water and pepper; simply set aside this mixture. Melt the butter in an ovenproof skillet on medium heat.

4. Transfer the onion and apple into the skillet to Sautee them until the onion is translucent. It takes around 5 to 6 minutes.

5. Place the onion and the apple mixture uniformly in the skillet.

6. Pour the mixture of eggs uniformly into the skillet, then simmer on medium heat till the sides are firm. Sprinkle some cheddar cheese at the end. Move the skillet into the oven and cook until the middle is firmly fixed. Around 12 to 15 minutes are required.

7. Break the omelet in half and move each half onto a single plate for serving.

32. Bagel with Salmon and Egg

|Calories:318| Total time: 15min | Servings: 1 | Difficulty: Easy

Ingredients

- Bagel, 1/2

- Cream cheese, 1 tablespoon

- Scallions, 1 tablespoon

- Fresh dill, 1/2 teaspoon

- Basil leaves, 2 fresh

- 1 sliced tomato

- Arugula, 4 pieces

- Egg 1 large

- Cooked salmon 1-ounce

Instruction

1. make two Slices of bagel toast, half of it in a toaster or microwave.

2. Chop the dill, basil leaves and scallions. Mix everything well with some cream and cheese.

3. Spread the mixture of cream cheese on previously toasted bagel halfway and use arugula and tomato slice for topping.

4. Start Heating the frying pan with a non-stick spray, coat it well and scramble the eggs.

5. Reheat the salmon using the same pan when the egg is being fried. Finally, on top of the tomato slice, place salmon and the egg and Enjoy it!

33. Cranberry Oatmeal Breakfast Cookies

|Calories:238 |Total time: 25min | Servings: 5 | Difficulty: Easy

Ingredients

- Unsalted butter, 1/2 cup

- Granulated sugar, 1/2 cup

- Egg 1 large

- All-purpose flour, 1/4 cup

- Vanilla extract, 1 teaspoon

- Cinnamon, 1/2 teaspoon

- Salt, 1/4 teaspoon

- Whey protein vanilla, 1.5 ounces

- Applesauce, 1 cup

- Rolled oats, 3 cups

- Dried cranberries, 1/2 cup

Instruction

1. start to melt the butter at room temperature.

2. Preheat the oven to 350degrees Fahrenheit Line the parchment paper in the oven with a baking sheet.

3. Mix the butter with sugar using an electric mixer.

4. Add the egg, rice, protein powder, salt, and cinnamon to the mixture.

5. Stir to blend. Add and mix apple sauce.

6. Then add oats and cranberries to the mixture.

7. Scoop out 1/4 cup scoops and put on the baking sheet. Slightly press the edges to flatten each cookie.

8. Bake until the cookies get golden brown color, but still tender, for 15 minutes. Allow cooling the cookies on the baking sheet for 5 minutes.

34. Festive Egg Scramble

|Calories:92 | Total time: 15min | Servings: 4 | Difficulty: Easy

Ingredients

- Egg substitute liquid (low cholesterol), 3-1/2 cups

- Onion, 1/2 cup

- Bell pepper red, 1/2 cup

- Bell pepper green, 1/2 cup

- Black pepper, 1 teaspoon

- Margarine (trans-fat free) 2 tablespoons

Instruction

1. Finely chop the onion and the bell pepper.

2. In a cup, mix egg product, bell pepper, onion, and black pepper.

3. in a pan, Melt the margarine

4. Add the egg product mixture and cook this mixture until the eggs have been set. Stir often to keep it from sticking.

5. Eat hot or when ready to serve.

35. Cheese with Grilled Corn Cakes

|Calories:285 |Total time: 10min | Servings: 4 | Difficulty: Easy

Ingredients

- White corn flour, 2/3 cup

- Crostino cheese, 4 ounces

- Anise, 1/2 teaspoon

- Hot water, 1 cup

- Butter, 1 teaspoon

Instruction

1. Put the corn-flour in the dish.

2. Melt the cheese, then add the anise with melted cheese to the starch.

3. Add some warm water, and blend well with the spatula.

4. Leave to sit for about 10 minutes and knead for 3 minutes.

5. Create 4 circles around 4-inch across and 1/2-inch thick for making the shape of the cakes.

6. Grease the butter pan or the saucepan pan.

7. Put each corn cake in a saucepan pan or skillet and cook them until they are lightly browned.

36. Fresh Spinach with Frittata

|Calories: 661 kcal |Total time: 45min | Servings: 4 | Difficulty: Easy

Ingredients

- Bacon 5 oz, diced

- Butter, 2 tablespoons

- Spinach, 8 oz, fresh

- Eggs 8

- Heavy whipping cream 1 cup

- Shredded cheese 5 oz

- Salt & pepper, as per taste

Directions

1. To 350 ° F preheat the oven. Grease individual ramekins or a 9x9 baking dish.

2. Fry the bacon over medium heat in butter till crispy. Add spinach and stir it until completely wilted. Remove the heated pan and set aside.

3. Whisk together the cream and eggs, then dump into ramekins or baking dish.

4. Cover with the bacon, cheese, and spinach and put it in the mid of the oven. Bake in the mid and on top golden brown for 25–30 mins, or until set.

37. Kidney friendly mushroom omelet

|Calories: 517 kcal |Total time: 15min | Servings: 4 | Difficulty: Easy

Ingredients

- Eggs, 3

- Butter, 1 oz

- Shredded cheese 1 oz

- Yellow onion, ¼, sliced

- Mushrooms, 4 larges, diced

- Salt & pepper, as per taste

Directions

1. Beat the eggs with a sprinkle of salt & pepper into a mixing cup. Whisk the eggs using a fork till smooth and shiny.

2. Melt the butter over med heat in a frying pan. Add the onion and mushrooms to the saucepan and cook until fresh. Then add in the mixture of the eggs around the vegetables.

3. Sprinkle cheese over the egg when the omelet starts to cook and get firm but has a bit raw egg on top.

4. Use a spatula to ease gently around the sides of the omelet, then turn it in half. From the heat, Remove the pan when it starts turning golden brown beneath, then transfers the omelet onto a tray.

38. Dilly scrambled eggs

|Calories: 229 kcal |Total time: 15min | Servings: 4 | Difficulty: Easy

Ingredients

- Butter, 1 oz

- Scallion 1, finely sliced

- Jalapeños 2, finely sliced and pickled

- Tomato, 1 finely sliced

- Eggs, 6

- Shredded cheese, 3 oz

- Salt & pepper, as per taste

Directions

1. Melt the butter in a wide frying pan over med-high heat.

2. Connect the scallions, tomatoes, and jalapeños, and fry for 3 to 4 minutes.

3. Beat the eggs and dump them into the saucepan. Scramble through for two min. Add seasonings and cheese.

---

39. Smoked Salmon Sandwich

|Calories: 556 kcal |Total time: 15min | Servings: 2 | Difficulty: Easy

Ingredients

pumpkin bread

- Pumpkin pie, 2 tablespoons

- Baking powder one tablespoon

- Salt, 1 teaspoon

- Husk powder ground psyllium, 2 tablespoons

- Flaxseed, ½ cup

- Almond flour, 1¼ cups

- Coconut flour, 1¼ cups

- Walnuts, 1⁄3 cup, chopped

- Pumpkin seeds, 1⁄3 cup plus for topping extra

- Eggs 3

- Apple sauce (unsweetened), ½ cup

- Coconut oil, ¼ cup

- Pumpkin puree, 14 oz

- Coconut oil, 1 tablespoon

Toppings

- Eggs 4

- Whipping cream, 2 tablespoons

- Butter, 2 oz, for frying

- Salt & pepper, as per taste

- Chili flakes, 1 pinch

- Butter, 2 tablespoons

- Leafy greens, 1 oz

- Salmon smoked 3 oz

Instructions

Pumpkin bread

1. To 200 ° C (400 ° F), Preheat the oven and grease 7-8 " bread pan with oil or butter.

2. Mix all the dry ingredients.

3. Bring the egg, pumpkin puree, apple sauce, and oil together and combine with the ingredients (dry) into a smooth mixture in a separate dish.

4. Pour in the dish (baking), then brush over a tablespoon of the pumpkin seeds.

5. Bake for one hour on the lower rack and take a toothpick to examine.

Sandwich

1. Whisk the eggs and the cream together. Garnish with salt & pepper.

2. Melt butter over med-high heat in the frying pan. Drop in the mixture of the eggs and stir till they blend and cook.

3. Stir in chili and blend. Using something you've dried chili flakes, tabasco, or new finely minced chili.

4. Toast the mild pumpkin bread, low-carb two pieces or the other low-carb loaf.

5. Put a dense Butter layer.

6. Place a couple of lettuce leaves on top and scrambled eggs, then incorporate the salmon and few finely minced chives.

40. Fried eggs, tomato, and cheese

|Calories: 417 kcal |Total time: 15min | Servings: 6/1 | Difficulty: Easy

Ingredients

- Eggs, 2

- Butter, ½ tablespoon

- Cheddar cheese, 2 oz, cubed

- Tomato, ½

- Black pepper & salt, ground

Instructions

1. Heat butter over medium heat in a frying pan.

2. Season the diced side of the tomato with salt & pepper. Put the tomato in a frying pan.

3. Break the eggs in the same pan. Leaving the eggs to scramble on one side for eggs sunny side up. Rotate the eggs for a couple of mins and cook for 1 more minute for eggs fried over quickly. Cook for a few more minutes for tougher yolks. Season with salt & pepper.

4. On a plate, Put the eggs, tomatoes, and cheese to eat. Scatter with dried oregano eggs and tomatoes for some additional flavor and taste.

5. A marinade.

6. Add the shrimp cubes and set it for some time and marinate for 5 minutes.

7. Heat the pan over low heat and add the marinade to the shrimp.

8. Stir-fry for 1 to 2 minutes before shrimp turns brown.

9. Take the pan from the fire and the spoon of the shrimp, leaving marinade.

10. Add the sour cream to the pan and swirl to blend.

11. Use a microwave or a skillet and heat tortillas.

12. Spread about 2 teaspoons of salsa over each tortilla. Cover with a mixture of 1/2 shrimp and scatter 1 tablespoon of cheese.

13. Add 1 tablespoon of the sour cream mixture on top of the shrimp. Now Fold the tortilla into half, change sides in the skillet, and extract from the pan.

14. Repeat the same process with the remaining tortilla and seafood, cheese, and marinade.

Chapter 2: Kidney Friendly Renal Diet Lunch Recipes

1. Brewery Burger

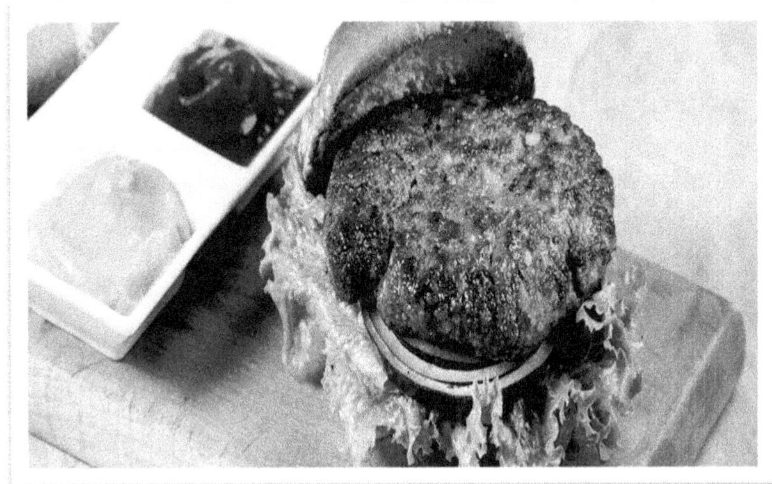

| Calories:242 | Total time: 25min | Servings: 4 | Difficulty: Easy

Ingredients

- Rice milk 3, tablespoons
- Soda crackers (salt-free), 5
- Egg, 1 large
- Herb seasoning salt-free (blend), 1 teaspoon
- 85% lean ground beef, 1-pound

Instruction

1. Crush down the soda crackers and mix with milk in a cup. Let them stay until the crackers become soft.
2. Beat the eggs and stir in a blend of crackers. Add the herb mixture; blend well if needed, dissolve the crackers. Add beef and blend properly.
3. Pat the beef mixture into four equal-sized patties.
4. Grill on moderate heat until the inside temperature is around 160 F.
5. Serve on the bun with the ideal toppings or serve the patty with the veggies and the starch of choice.

2. Chicken Pita Pizza BBQ

|Calories:320 | Total time: 25min | Servings: 2 | Difficulty: Easy

Ingredients

- 6-1/2" size pita bread, 2

- Barbecue sauce (low sodium), 3 tablespoons

- Purple onion, 1/4 cup

- Crumbled feta cheese, 2 tablespoons

- Chicken, cooked, 4 ounces

- Garlic powder, 1/8 teaspoon

Instruction

1. Preheat the oven to 350 degrees F.

2. Spray the non-stick cooking oil on the baking sheet and put 2 pitas on the sheet.

3. Spread about 1-1/2 tablespoon of BBQ sauce (low sodium) on each pita.

4. Chop the onion and sprinkle it over pitas.

5. Make Cubs of chicken and scatter over the pitas.

6. Sprinkle some feta cheese along with garlic powder over the pitas.

7. Bake for 13 minutes.

8. Serve hot.

3. Crunchy Chicken Wraps

|Calories:260| Total time: 25min | Servings: 4 | Difficulty: Easy

Ingredients

- Stalk celery, 1

- Medium carrot, 1

- Bell pepper red, 1/2

- Mayonnaise low-fat, 1/4 cup

- Onion powder, 1/2 teaspoon

- Wheat lavash whole 2

- Canned chicken (low sodium), 8 ounces

Instruction

1. start by dicing carrot, celery, and bell pepper.

2. In a medium cup, add the mayonnaise and mix it with onion powder.

3. Spread 2 teaspoons of this mixture on every lavash flatbread.

4. Mix all diced vegetables in a different dish.

5. Put four ounces of chicken with half of the diced vegetables on one side of each slice of flatbread.

6. Roll up the side of flatbread and split the diagonal of flatbread in half. Now secure each half of it with the help of a toothpick.

7. Protect half of each tortilla using a toothpick and split each tortilla wrap in half.

4. Shrimp Quesadilla

|Calories:318| Total time: 15min | Servings: 2 | Difficulty: Easy

Ingredients

- Raw shrimp, 5 ounces

- Cilantro, 2 tablespoons

- Lemon juice, 1 tablespoon

- Ground cumin, 1/4 teaspoon

- Cayenne pepper, 1/8 teaspoon

- Burrito size flour tortillas 2

- Sour cream, 2 tablespoons

- Salsa, 4 teaspoons

- Cheddar cheese, shredded jalapeno, 2 tablespoons

Instruction

1. Rinse Shell and shrimp and break into pieces of bite-size. Chop the coriander.

2. In a zip-lock pack, add lemon juice, cilantro, cayenne pepper and cumin to create a marinade.

3. Add the shrimp cubes and set it for some time and marinate for 5 minutes.

4. Heat the pan over low heat and add the marinade to the shrimp.

5. Stir-fry for 1 to 2 minutes before shrimp turns brown.

6. Take the pan from the fire and the spoon of the shrimp, leaving marinade.

7. Add the sour cream to the pan and swirl to blend.

8. Use a microwave or a skillet and heat tortillas.

9. Spread about 2 teaspoons of salsa over each tortilla. Cover with a mixture of 1/2 shrimp and scatter 1 tablespoon of cheese.

10. Add 1 tablespoon of the sour cream mixture on top of the shrimp. Now Fold the tortilla into half, change sides in the skillet, and extract from the pan.

11. Repeat the same process with the remaining tortilla and seafood, cheese, and marinade.

12. Break the tortilla into 4 bits. Garnish with some cilantro and lemon wedge if ready to eat.

5. Mexican Seasoning with Soft Tacos

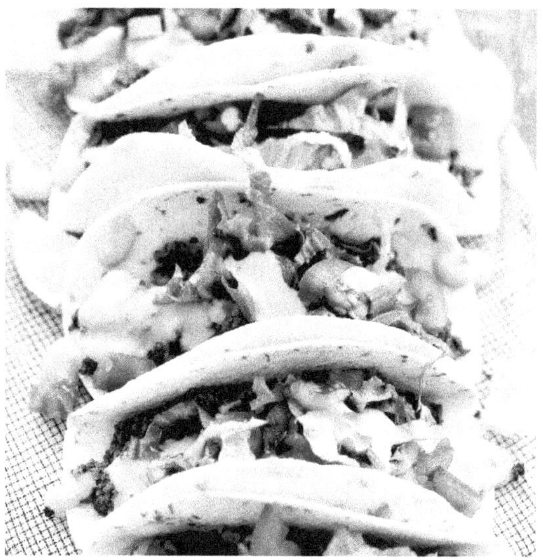

|Calories:340 |Total time: 15min | Servings: 7 | Difficulty: Easy

Ingredients

- Onion, 5 tablespoons

- Lettuce, 2 cups

- Ground beef, 1-pound

- Tomato sauce low-sodium, 1/2 cup

- 6-inch flour tortillas, 14

- Shredded cheddar cheese, 5 tablespoons

- Sour cream, 5 tablespoons

Instruction

1. Chop the lettuce and the onion together.

2. Brown the meat and allow to rinse

3. Add the spices and the mixture of low-sodium sauce.

4. Heat on medium flame. Heat the tortillas.

5. To produce soft tacos, take one flour tortilla, then add 1/4 cup of cooked ground beef; after that, add 1 Teaspoon of cheese, 1 Teaspoon of onion, 1 Teaspoon of sour cream and finally lettuce as needed.

6. Enjoy it.

6. Tortilla Beef Rollups

|Calories:258|Total time: 15min | Servings: 2 | Difficulty: Easy

Ingredients

- 6" size flour tortilla,

- Whipped cheese cream, 2 tablespoons

- Roast beef, (cooked), 5 ounces

- Chopped red onion, 1/4 cup

- Bell pepper cut in slices red, yellow, or green, 1/4

- Cucumber slices, 8

- Lettuce leaves romaine, 2

- Mrs. Dash seasoning herb blend, 1 teaspoon

Instruction

1. Layer the cheese cream over the tortilla.

2. Divide the mixture in half to produce two tortillas.

3. Place a layer of red onion, roast beef, bell pepper slices, cucumbers slices and lettuce on each the tortilla

4. Sprinkle some Mrs. Dash herb seasoning over it.

5. Roll it up, such as a jellyroll.

6. Break the tortilla into 4 parts or serve the entire tortilla.

7. Chicken Noodle Soup

|Calories:186| Total time: 30min | Servings: 6 | Difficulty: Easy

Ingredients

- Unsalted Butter, 1 tablespoon

- Chopped Onions, 1/2 cup

- Chopped Celery, 1/2 cup

- Chicken Stock, 5 cups

- Cooked Chicken Breast, 8 ounces

- Egg Noodles Dry, 2 cups

- Sliced Carrots, 1 cup

- Ground Basil, 1/2 Teaspoon

- Ground Oregano, 1/2 Teaspoon

- Ground Black Pepper, 1/4 Teaspoon

Instruction

1. First of all, roast all the chicken and cut it into tiny bits.

2. Wash and wipe all your vegetables.

3. In a 5-quarter Dutch oven, on medium heat, melt the butter.

4. Cook the onion and celery with butter until it becomes tender; about 5 minutes are enough.

5. Add chicken stock and mix in chicken, pasta, carrots, basil, oregano, and pepper. Get things to a simmer. Reduce heat and boil for 20 minutes.

6. Serve it. Allows 6 servings, and roughly 2 cups equate to 1 meal.

---

8. Asian Pear Crisp

|Calories:401 | Total time: 60min | Servings: 6 | Difficulty: Easy

Ingredients

- Chopped nuts, 3/4 cup

- All-purpose flour unbleached, 1/2 cup

- Light brown sugar, 1/4 cup

- Granulated sugar, 4 tablespoons

- Ground cinnamon, 1/4 teaspoon

- Ground nutmeg, 1/8 teaspoon

- Unsalted butter, 5 tablespoons

- Cornstarch, 1 tablespoon

- One lemon juice

- Peeled & cored, Asian pears 3 pounds,

Instruction

1. Preheat the oven to 370 °.

2. In the food processor, combine almonds, flour, brown sugar, 2 teaspoons of granulated sugar, some cinnamon and nutmeg.

3. Pour the molten butter over the mixture and blend until the mixture appears like wet powder.

4. In a wide cup, whisk the remaining 2 teaspoons of granulated sugar with cornstarch and lemon juice.

5. Peel the pears, make half the heart. Split them in wedges and cut it in half.

6. Mix the pears with a combination of sugar and move to an 8" square baking dish.

7. Sprinkle as topping on the pears.

8. Bake until the fruit bursts around the edges and the topping get golden. It takes around 45 minutes.

9. Cool on the wire rack for about 15 minutes. Then Serve it.

9. Asian Pear Torte

|Calories:426|Total time: 40min | Servings: 8 | Difficulty: Easy

Ingredients

- Almonds, 1 1/2 cups plus 1/4 cup for garnishing

- Flour, 1 1/2 cups

- Sugar, 2/3 cup

- Lemon zest, 1 tablespoon

- Cinnamon, 1 teaspoon

- Almond extract, 1 teaspoon

- Cold unsalted butter 1 cup, cut into cubes

- Yolks, 2 egg

- Asian pears, 2-3

- Apple, 1/2 cup, lemon marmalade or currant jelly

- Powdered sugar and maraschino cherry for garnish

Instruction

1. Preheat the oven to 375 degrees.

2. Use a food processor, and add 1 1⁄2 cups of almonds, rice, butter, lemon, and cinnamon till the nuts become finely chopped.

3. Add the extract of almonds, butter, and egg yolks.

4. Pulse on to blend. Grease the surface and sides of the 9" spring pan after filling with the batter, pressing to the edges. Reserve 1/4-1/2 cup of the batter for later.

5. Cut Asian Pears into 1/4" wide slices.

6. Starting in the middle of the batter, add layer of slices in consecutive rings. Make two full rings across the top of the cake.

7. Spread the batter kept for reserve over the side of the cake and the end of slices of pears to create a crust type.

8. Melt the jelly using a microwave for 1 minute, then brush the Asian pear slices.

9. Sprinkle almonds on the edges and in the middle.

10. Bake for 30-35 minutes.

11. Let it cool before opening the spring pan.

12. Garnish it with maraschino cherry and dust it with some powdered sugar.

10. Baked Potato Soup

|Calories:216| Total time: 30min | Servings: 6 | Difficulty: Easy

Ingredients

- Potatoes large 2

- Flour, 1/3 cup

- Skim milk, 4 cups

- Pepper, 1/2 teaspoon

- Shredded low fat jack cheese, 4 ounces

- Sour cream no fat, 1/2 cup

Instruction

1. Bake the potatoes at 400 ° until soft.

2. Let them cool for a while.

3. Break them lengthwise and scoop out all the pulp.

4. Place the flour in a wide saucepan. Gradually add milk and stir until mixed.

5. Add the pulp and then pepper to the mix.

6. Cook on medium heat until it becomes thick and bubbles are produced. Stir continuously.

7. Add butter, whisk until the cheese is molten.

8. Turn off the heat and stir in some sour cream.

11. BBQ Winter Squash

|Calories:99g|Total time: 25min | Servings: 2 | Difficulty: Easy

Ingredients

- Sliced butternut squash 1-2 acorn, 1" thick slices

- Olive oil, 1-2 tablespoons

- Brown sugar, 1-2 tablespoons

- Butter, 1-2 tablespoons

Instruction

1. Heat the grill (about 400 degrees).

2. Brush the squash with a thin layer of olive oil and put on the grill for around five min and turn.

3. When the fork is tender, brush with some amount of melted butter and brown sugar.

4. Leave to the grill for 1 minute, then remove and serve.

12. Beef Barley Soup

|Calories:270 | Total time: 2hour | Servings: 6 | Difficulty: Easy

Ingredients

- Black pepper, 1/2 teaspoon

- Diced 1-inch cubes of stew beef meat, 2 lbs.

- Vegetable oil, 1/4 cup

- Chopped onion, 1 cup

- Sliced mushrooms, 1/2 cup

- Diced carrots, 2

- Minced garlic, 1/2 teaspoon

- Dried thyme, 1/4 teaspoon

- Low sodium chicken broth, 1 can (14.5 ounces)

- Water, 3 cups

- 1 frozen package of vegetables (16 ounces)

- Soaked and diced potatoes, 2

- Barley, 1/2 cup

Instruction

1. Season the beef with some pepper.

2. Add 2 teaspoons of oil to the pot and sauté for 5 minutes.

3. Add 2 more teaspoons of oil to add the onion, carrots, and mushrooms.

4. Sauté for 5 minutes while stirring regularly.

5. Add garlic and thyme and sauté for 3 minutes.

6. Add the chicken and the water to the pot.

7. Add the mixed vegetables, the beans, and the barley.

8. Stir in and put to a simmer.

9. Cover and lower the heat.

10. Simmer for 1 to 1 1/2 hours.

13. Beef or Chicken Enchiladas

|Calories:235| Total time: 30min| Servings: 5 | Difficulty: Easy

Ingredients

- Lean ground beef or chicken, 1-pound

- Onion chopped, 1/2 cup

- Cumin, 1 teaspoon

- Black pepper, 1/2 teaspoon

- Chopped garlic clove, 1

- Corn tortillas 12

- Enchilada sauce, 1 can

Instruction

5. Preheat the oven to 375 °.

6. Brown beef in a frying pan.

7. Add the onion, some garlic, cumin, and pepper as per taste. Keep cooking. Stir until the onion becomes soft.

8. Fry tortillas with some oil in another skillet.

9. Dip through salsa of enchilada each tortilla

10. Fill the beef mixture, then roll it up.

11. Put the enchilada in a small pan and if needed, cover with sauce and the cheese.

12. Bake until the cheese has melted, and the enchiladas are golden colored.

13. Finished with whipped cream, put sliced olives over or other toppings of your choice.

14. Biscuits with Master Mix

|Calories:174 | Total time: 20min | Servings:6 | Difficulty: Easy

Ingredients

- Master Mix, 3 cups

- Water, 2/3 cup

Instruction

1. Preheat the oven to 450 ° f.

2. Mix the products and blend properly.

3. Let it settle for 5 minutes.

4. Knead the dough around 15 times on a lightly floured surface.

5. Roll out around 1/2-inch thickness, then cut with the help of a floured cutter until 12 biscuits are made

6. Place them 2 inches apart from each other on a non-greased baking sheet.

7. Bake for 12-15 minutes or until golden brown.

15. Black-Eyed Peas

|Calories:130|Total time: 1.5hour | Servings: 6 | Difficulty: Easy

Ingredients

- Dried Black-eyed peas, 2 cups

- Water or vegetable stock (low sodium) 3 1/2 cups

- Smoked turkey (optional), 12 ounces

- Finely chopped onion medium size, 1

- Finely chopped garlic cloves 5 to 6

- Diced celery, 1 cup

- Thyme, 1/2 teaspoon

- Ginger, 1/2 teaspoon

- Curry powder, 1/2 teaspoon

- Cayenne pepper, 1 pinch

Instruction

1. using a wide bowl, add the black-eyed peas, then add approximately 4 inches of water.

2. Cover and allow to soak for about 6 hours or overnight.

3. Rinse the peas and clean under cool water.

4. Add the black-eyed peas and the remaining ingredients to a big jar.

5. Bring to a boil and reduce heat to medium, cover with a solid lid and simmer until peas get soft, which will take around 1 1/2 hours.

6. Stir occasionally.

16. Blasted Brussels Sprouts

|Calories:68 |Total time: 25min | Servings: 4| Difficulty: Easy

Ingredients

- Brussels Sprouts, 2 cups (one stalk)

- olive oil, 1-2 tablespoons

- fresh Cheese grated Parmesan, 2-4 tablespoons

- flavored vinegar fruit or herb, 1/4 cup

Instruction

1. Preheat the oven to 450 ° f.

2. Clean the leaves.

3. Break the bigger sprouts in half leave the smaller sprouts intact.

4. Simply mix the olive oil with the sprouts.

5. Place them on a lightly oiled baking sheet.

6. Roast for approximately 10 minutes. The Sprouts are considered to be done and tender when pierced with a fork.

7. Take out from the oven, then sprinkle some fruit vinegar and add fresh Parmesan cheese.

17. Broccoli Chicken Casserole

|Calories:368| Total time: 1.5hour | Servings: 6 | Difficulty: Easy

Ingredients

- Cooked broccoli, 2-3 cups

- Chopped onion, 1 medium size

- Diced chicken breast, 2-3

- Butter or margarine, 2 tablespoons

- Beaten eggs, 2

- Milk, 2 cups

- Cooked rice, 2 cups barley, or noodles

- Grated cheese, 2 cups

- Grated parmesan for garnishing

Instruction

1. Preheat the oven to 350°.

2. Use microwave and put the broccoli in it, now cover with the plastic wrap and cook in microwave until bright green. It takes around 2-3 minutes.

3. In the meanwhile, cook the onions until they get brown add chicken with honey.

4. Mix all ingredients and place in a greased saucepan.

5. Sprinkle some grated parmesan on the top, then bake for around 1.5 hours or until fully set and fork passes through.

18. Brown Bag Popcorn

|Calories:155|Total time: 4min | Servings: 1 | Difficulty: Easy

Ingredients

- Popcorn kernels, 1/4 cup

- Canola oil, 1 teaspoon

- Lunch bag brown paper, 1

Instruction

1. add popcorn and a little amount of oil in a wide bowl.

2. Place the popcorns in a brown sack, close the top and staple the close edge twice.

3. Use microwave and place in it for 3 minutes or till there is some kind of popping sound is heard.

19. Burritos Rapidos

|Calories:232| Total time: 10min | Servings: 4 | Difficulty: Easy

Ingredients

- Olive or canola oil, 1 1/2 teaspoons

- Diced bell pepper, red 1/2

- Thin slices of onions (scallions), green4

- Beaten eggs, 8

- Corn tortillas, (6-inch) 4

Instruction

1. Heat the oil in a medium-size frying pan over medium heat.

2. Add the bell pepper and the green onion and roast for around 3 minutes or until softened.

3. Add the eggs, then scramble for about five min or until the eggs are completely cooked.

4. Place tortillas between the two wet towel papers and place them on a tray.

5. Finally, Microwave tortillas for two minutes.

6. Spoon the egg mixture to the hot tortillas.

7. Roll up these tortillas and enjoy yourself.

8. Try applying a splash of hot sauce and sprinkle some chili powder for a slightly rich taste.

20. Buttermilk Ranch Dressing

|Calories:83g| Total time: 30min | Servings: 2 | Difficulty: Easy

Ingredients

- Mayonnaise, 1/2 cup

- Milk, 1/2 cup

- Vinegar, 2 tablespoons

- Chopped fresh chives, 1 tablespoon

- Dill, 1 tablespoon

- Chopped oregano leaves, 1 tablespoon

- Garlic powder, 1/4 teaspoon

Instruction

1. In a medium cup, whisk the mayonnaise with cream and vinegar.

2. Add fresh chips with dill, oregano leaves and 1/4 teaspoon of garlic powder.

3. Mix it.

4. Chill for at least 1 hour to encourage the flavors to mature.

5. Stir in the dressing just before eating.

21. Canned Fish Tacos

|Calories:155| Total time: 10min | Servings: 2 | Difficulty: Easy

Ingredients

- Chopped onion, 2 tablespoons

- Oil, 2 teaspoons

- Tuna rinsed, 1 can

- Canned or frozen corn, 1/2 cup

- Diced canned tomatoes, 1/4 cup without salt

- Chili powder, 1/2 teaspoon

- Corn tortillas, 4

Instruction

1. Use a frying pan and cook the onion with the oil over medium flame until onions become clear in color.

2. Add fish, maize, tomatoes, and chili powder.

3. Cook until it is heated throughout, around 3-5 minutes.

4. Serve with some soft tortillas. If needed, Add sour cream it and lettuce with hot sauce.

5. You can swap canned tuna with canned salmon. If not, then chicken may be used. You may consider using 1/2 Teaspoon of onion powder instead of fresh onion.

22. Carrot Muffins

|Calories:206 |Total time: 30min | Servings: 8 | Difficulty: Easy

Ingredients

- All-purpose flour, 1/2 cup

- Whole wheat flour, 1/2 cup

- Oats, 1/2 cup

- Ground flaxseed, 1/4 cup optional

- Baking powder, 3/4 teaspoon

- Baking soda, 3/4 teaspoon

- Cinnamon, 3/4 teaspoon

- Ginger (optional) ,1/2 teaspoon

- Brown sugar, 1/2 cup

- Vegetable oil, 1/2 cup

- Eggs, 2 larges

- Unsweetened applesauce, 1/2 cup

- Fresh ginger (optional), 2-inch piece

- Shredded carrots (~6 medium sizes) 2 cups

Instruction

1. Preheat the oven to 350 °

2. Coat the muffin tins slightly with some oil or non-stick spray.

3. Mix the dry ingredients in a large bowl.

4. Use a fork or whisk to combine the moist ingredients in a medium dish.

5. Stir the wet ingredients into the dry ingredients before they are mixed.

6. Add in shredded carrots meanwhile, stir occasionally

7. Cover the muffins with the batter evenly.

8. Bake for approximately 20 minutes.

23. Corn and Chicken Chowder

Calories:472 |Total time: 32min | Servings: 6 | Difficulty: Easy

Ingredients

- Bacon (low sodium), 12 slices

- Chopped onions, 2

- Low sodium chicken broth, 7 cups

- Diced and soaked potatoes, 4

- Corn, 8 cups

- Diced chicken breasts boneless, 8

- Fresh chopped thyme, 6 tablespoons

- Mocha mix, 4 cups

- black pepper, 1/2 teaspoon

- Green chopped onions, 8

Instruction

1. Cook the bacon in the skillet until it is crisply cut the bacon and put aside.

2. Sautee the slices of onions in the fat of the bacon

3. Add the butter and the potatoes.

4. Cover and cook for 10 minutes.

5. Add some maize, chicken, and thyme.

6. Now Cover and boil till the chicken is cooked; it will take around 15 minutes.

7. Mix in the broth and boil for 2 minutes.

8. Sprinkle with sausage, pepper, and some green onions.

24. Chicken and Dumplings

|Calories:401 |Total time: 8hour | Servings: 6 | Difficulty: Easy

Ingredients

- Whole chicken, 1 or chopped chicken, 3 lbs.

- Chicken broth or, 2 cups of water

- Finely cut celery leaves, 1 stalk

- Sliced carrots, 2-3

- Black pepper, 1/2 teaspoon

- Mace or nutmeg, 1/2 teaspoon

- 1/4 cup flour

- Eggs, 2

- Milk, 2/3 cup

- Baking powder, 3 teaspoons

- Flour, 2 cups

- Margarine or unsalted butter, 2 tablespoons

Instruction

1. Put chicken and vegetables with some spices, then add water or chicken broth in a cooker.

2. Add more water, sufficient to cover the chicken with around 1".

3. Put the cooker on slow heat for around 6-8 hours.

4. Put the chicken in the ovenproof bowl.

5. If you like, then remove the bones, or they may just fall off automatically.

6. Cover and keep it warm.

7. Turn the cooker heat to high. Now add 1/4 cup of flour and whisk rapidly to prevent lumps.

8. Break the butter into 2 cups with a knife.

9. Mix the wet ingredients for a stiff dough and add a spoon of boiling broth.

10. Cover the pot, reduce the heat to stop boiling, now cook slowly for 15 mins without removing the cap.

11. Place chicken inside a large serving dish then pours over the thickened sauce. Serve with dumplings.

25. Chicken Lasagna and White Sauce

|Calories:453| Total time: 60min | Servings: 6 | Difficulty: Easy

Ingredients

- Chicken breast or thigh, 6 oz.

- Chicken broth 12 ounces low sodium

- Olive oil, 1/4 cup

- Diced onion, 1 large

- Oregano, 1 tablespoon

- Black pepper, 1/4 teaspoon

- White wine (optional), 1/4 cup

- Thick-sliced mushrooms, 1/2 cup

- Flour, 3 tablespoons

- Cream cheese, 6 ounces

- Mocha mix, 1 1/2 cups

- Nutmeg, 1/4-1/2 teaspoon

- Fresh parmesan cheese, grated 1/2 cup

- Sliced into little moons, 1 1/2 zucchini,

- Lasagna noodles not boiled, 1 package

Instruction

1. Preheat oven to 325 F.

2. Put chicken and stock in a small pan, then bring to a boil, now reduce heat and simmer once chicken becomes white and thoroughly cooked. The chicken cooks

    better if it is sliced into bits.

3. In the meantime, add some olive oil, oregano with onions, then add black pepper in a wide saucepan over medium heat, Now sauté everything for 5 min or until the onion starts to soften.

4. Add to the pan some wine and encourage to evaporate it.

5. Add the mushrooms.

6. Sprinkle the flour evenly over the plate, mixing slightly to scatter the flavors.

7. Now on low heat, cook about 3 minutes

8. Split the cream cheese and return it to the pan, stirring it again until it is melted and uniformly spread. (~2 min.)

9. Slowly add the Mocha mixture to the plate, stirring again.

10. Ingredients should now be thickening, not clumpy. If it is all clumpy, carry on stirring to split them up.

11. Add some nutmeg.

12. Stir in now parmesan cheese and keep stirring while it heats for another 5 mins. The sauce must also be thickened.

13. Take the chicken out from the pot (save the broth), use two knives, break the chicken and attempt to hold the bits intact.

14. Put it aside. Stir in half a cup of the remaining broth into the cream mixture while stirring regularly for 2 minutes.

15. Put the lasagna sheets on the pan, cover with 1/3 sauce, add 1/2 of the chicken with 1/2 of the parts of the zucchini, spread thinly on top.

16. Cover with foil, put it in the oven for around 30 minutes and cut the foil before crisp.

26. Chicken Seafood Gumbo

|Calories:240|Total time: 45min | Servings:6 | Difficulty: Easy

Ingredients

- Canola oil, 1 tablespoon
- Chopped celery stalks, 3
- Chopped yellow onion, 1
- Chopped bell pepper red, 1
- Chopped chicken breasts skinless, 2
- Sliced lean smoked turkey sausage 8 ounces,
- Canola oil, 1/2 cup
- Flour, 1/2 cup
- Cajun seasoning salt-free, 1 tablespoon
- Chicken broth low sodium 2 quarts
- Cooked shrimp, 1/2 pound
- Canned crab, 6 ounces
- Chopped frozen okra, 3 cups

Instruction

1. Heat about 1 tablespoon of canola oil in 4.5-quarter or a larger pot over medium heat.
2. Add the celery, cabbage, clove pepper with chicken and sausage and simmer for about 10 minutes.
3. Take the mixture out of the pot and put it aside.
4. Decrease the heat to medium.
5. Now add about 1/2 cup of canola oil, then add some flour to make the roux.
6. Stir in the Cajun seasoning and simmer for 1 minute or more it depends on how much dark you like.
7. Slowly mix in chicken broth while constantly stirring to prevent lumps.
8. Increase the heat to medium level and allow the mixture to boil for around 10 minutes or before it begins to thicken slightly.

9. Reduce heat now to medium and then add crabs, okra, and chicken mixture back to the pot.

10. Cook for about 10 minutes or until the mixture is properly heated

27. Cornbread Stuffing with Chicken

|Calories:372| Total time: 1.5hour | Servings: 4 | Difficulty: Easy

Ingredients

- Fresh parsley, 1 tablespoon

- 2 tablespoons, Dash (original blend) + 1 1/2 teaspoons extra

- Mrs. Dash (chicken grilling blend), 1 tablespoon

- Skinless boneless, chicken breast, 4 (4 ounces) pieces

- Unsalted butter, 1 tablespoon

- Chopped celery, 1 cup

- Chopped onion, 1/2 cup

- Ground sage, 2 teaspoons

- Coarsely crumbled cornbread, 2 cups (about 7 ounces)

- Unseasoned croutons, 2 cups

- chicken broth (low sodium), 1 cup

Instruction

1. Chop the parsley.

2. Mix 1 tablespoon of Mrs. Dash® (Original Blend) with Mrs. Dash® (Chicken Grilling Blend) and parsley.

3. Cover chicken breasts from all sides with a blend of seasoning.

4. Spray on a large non-stick stove some cooking spray.

5. Heat the skillet over medium flame until it is hot.

6. Add the chicken breasts to the skillet, cook for 3 to 5 min each side or until lightly golden.

7. Take the chicken breasts from the skillet and put them aside.

8. Preheat the oven to 35F.

9. Melt the butter in a saucepan over low heat. Add the celery, the cabbage, 1 tablespoon + 1 1/2 Teaspoon of Mrs. Dash® (Original Blend), the sage, and the combination.

10. Cook over medium heat for 6-7 minutes or until all vegetables are soft.

11. Remove from the heat.

12. In a mixing dish, combine the cornbread crumbs and croutons.

13. Add the mixture of vegetables and the broth by swirling to combine.

14. Spoon the dressing mixture on a large baking dish lightly coated with some non-stick cooking oil.

15. Organize chicken breasts with dressing mixture.

16. Cover and bake at 350 ° for 45 minutes.

17. Remove cover and continue cooking for 5 minutes or till the chicken breast's internal temperature is around 170 degrees.

18. Garnish using leaves of celery, if needed.

28. Cider Cream Chicken

|Calories:186|Total time: 30min | Servings:6min | Difficulty: Easy

Ingredients

- Chicken breasts, 4 (bones in)

- Unsalted butter, 2 tablespoons

- Apple cider, 3/4 cup

Instruction

1. Melt the butter over medium heat. Add chicken and make it brown from all sides.

2. Add the cider and decrease the heat to medium flame; boil for around 20 minutes.

3. Remove the chicken from the skillet.

4. Boil the cider until it is reduced to around 1/4 cup.

5. Put in the cream sauce over the chicken and eat.

---

29. Collard Greens

|Calories:50 |Total time: 30min | Servings:4 | Difficulty: Easy

Ingredients

- Olive oil, 1 1/2 teaspoons

- Chopped onion, 1/2

- Minced garlic, 2 teaspoons

- Collard greens, 1 large bunch, (stems removed)

- Black pepper, 1/8 teaspoon

- Red pepper flakes, 1/2 teaspoon

- Fat-free chicken broth (low-sodium), 1 to 1 1/2 cups

- Vinegar, 2 tablespoons

Instruction

1. Heat the oil over medium-high heat, then add onions and garlic, now cook the mixture until it becomes soft (but do not burn).

2. Add about 1/4 of the vegetables and mix with garlic and onion.

3. When the vegetables are wilted, add the remaining vegetables in the batches before they are wilted. Mix with black pepper some red pepper flakes.

4. Add the broth to get it to a simmer.

5. Reduce heat and boil for around 20 minutes or until soft. The broth should now be completely reduced

6. Remove from flame and pour on the vinegar before eating.

---

30. Confetti Chicken Rice

|Calories:519| Total time: 40min | Servings: 4 | Difficulty: Easy

Ingredients

- Olive oil, 3 tablespoons
- Skinless, boneless, chicken breast 1 piece
- About 2 1/4 cups non-salted frozen corn
- Cubes of, 1 fresh zucchini
- Cubed bell pepper red, 1 large
- Red diced onion medium size, 1
- Garlic powder, 1/2 teaspoon
- Cumin, 1 tablespoon
- Black pepper, 1/2 teaspoon
- Mrs. Dash (original blend), 2 teaspoons
- Cayenne pepper, 1/4 teaspoon
- Original ready rice (uncle ben's), 1 package

Instruction

1. Use a large non-stick skillet, and heat 2 tablespoons of olive oil over medium-high heat.
2. When the oil gets hot, put the chicken breast over the hot skillet carefully.
3. When the juice evaporates, extract the chicken from the skillet (about 15 minutes are required).
4. Add 1 tablespoon of olive oil to the same skillet, add zucchini, corn, onions, and red pepper.
5. Sautee on low to medium heat and cook till onions start to soften (about 10 minutes).
6. Then add the garlic powder, the cumin, the black pepper, Mrs. Dash, and the cayenne pepper.
7. Revert the chicken to skillet, now lower the heat to medium and whisk the mixture for around 5 minutes.
8. Follow the guidelines on the box of rice.
9. Add all the rice into the cooked vegetables and begin sautéing for a couple of more

minutes.

10. Serve hot.

---

31. Alaska Baked Macaroni and Cheese

|Calories:424 |Total time: 30min | Servings: 6| Difficulty: Easy

Ingredients

- Bowtie pasta or small shell, 3 cups

- Flour, 2 tablespoons

- Unsalted butter, 2 tablespoons

- Milk, 2 cups

- Mustard powder, 1 teaspoon

- Paprika, 1 teaspoon

- Fresh thyme, 1 tablespoon or chopped tarragon, 1 teaspoon

- Cheese, 2 cups

- Croutons or almonds as per taste

Instruction

1. Heat the oven to 350 °.

2. Boil the pasta in a big pot until settled

3. Measure both the flour and butter in a medium measuring glass cup. Microwave for around 1-2 minutes until it becomes golden brown.

4. Slowly stir in the milk and begin to microwave until thickened. Now Stir in the herbs and all spices.

5. Mix the drained pasta, sauce with cheese, and put them in a baking dish (greased). Bake for approximately 20 minutes.

6. Before the last 5 minutes, finish by topping with croutons or sliced almonds.

32. Almond Pecan Caramel Corn

|Calories: 300 |Total time: 1hour | Servings:5 | Difficulty: Easy

Ingredients

- Popped popcorn 20 cups or popcorn kernels about, 3/4 cup

- Almonds 2 cups, unblenched

- Pecan halves, 1 cup

- Sugar 1 cup, ground

- Butter 1 cup, unsalted

- Corn syrup, 1/2 cup

- Cream of tartar a pinch

- Baking soda, 1 teaspoon

Instruction

1. In a broad fry pan, layer cooked popcorn uniformly with almonds as well as pecans.

2. In a big heavy saucepan, mix sugar, tartar cream, butter, and corn syrup.

3. Bring it to boil under a medium-high flame, stirring continuously. Let it simmer for

1. about five minutes without stirring.

4. Remove the heat, then stir in the baking soda mixture.

5. Pour caramel generously over a mixture of popcorn, swirling to cover properly.

6. Bake for about 1 hour at 200°, swirling after 10 minutes.

7. Let it cool, stirring often. Store in a sealed tin for about a week.

33. Apple Bran Muffins

|Calories: 234 |Total time: 1hour | Servings: 8 | Difficulty: Easy

Ingredients

- Wheat flour, 2 cups, whole

- Wheat bran, 1 1/2 cups

- Baking soda, 1 1/4 teaspoons

- Nutmeg, 1/2 teaspoon

- Orange rind, 1 tablespoon, grated

- Apple, 1 cup, sliced

- Raisins, 1/2 cup

- Nuts or sunflower seeds 1/2 cup, sliced

- Orange juice (from 1 orange)

- Buttermilk or sour milk scant, 2 cups

- Egg 1, beaten

- Molasses, 1/2 cup

- Oil, 2 tablespoons

Instruction

1. Preheat the oven to 350 degrees.

2. Blend flour, bran, soda as well as nutmeg along with a fork.

3. Mix it in the orange rind, the apples, raisins, nuts as well as seeds.

4. Take the juice of one orange into 2 cups, then add the buttermilk in it to make 2

5. cups.

6. Blend buttermilk mixture, eggs, molasses, and oil together and stir thoroughly.

7. Stir the liquid ingredients into the dry ingredients in few quick strokes.

8. Now pour it into oiled muffin tins, then fill them with two-thirds of the mixture,

9. and bake for about 25 minutes.

34. Alfredo Sauce

|Calories: 73 Total time: 10min | Servings: 6 | Difficulty: Easy

Ingredients

- Olive oil, 1/4 cup

- All-purpose flour, 3 tablespoons

- Garlic 1 clove, crushed

- Rice milk, 2 cups

- Cream cheese, 4 ounces

- Parmesan cheese, 1/3 cup, shredded

- Nutmeg 1/4 teaspoon, crushed

- Lemon juice, 1 tablespoon

Instruction

1. Take olive oil inside a large saucepan and heat it over medium flame. Add the

1. flour, then whisk it to the paste and then add the chopped garlic.

2. Gradually add rice milk, constantly stirring to avoid lumps. Let the mixture boil

3. as well as thicken.

4. Add the cream cheese and stir well. Remove the heat.

5. Add 1/3 cup of Parmesan cheese, nutmeg as well as lemon juice. Now mix well.

6. Serve with spaghetti, chicken, steamed tomatoes, etc.

35. Apple and Cream Cheese Torte

|Calories: 298 Total time: 55min | Servings: 6 | Difficulty: Easy

Ingredients

- Butter, 1/2 cup, unsalted and softened

- Sugar, 3/4 cup, separated into 1/4 cups

- Flour, 1 cup

- Cream cheese 8 ounces, softened

- Egg, 1

- Vanilla, 1 teaspoon

- Apples 3-4 medium, finely diced

* Cinnamon, 1/2 teaspoon

Instruction

1. Pre-heat the oven to 450 °.

2. Take cream butter with 1/4 cup of sugar and blend them with flour in a medium bowl.

3. Now press them into a spring shape pan.

4. Take cream cheese, sugar about (1/4 cup), one egg, and vanilla, then beat them until smooth.

5. Spread it in the spring shape pan.

6. Add the rest of the 1/4 cup of sugar and cinnamon and mix them with apples.

7. Arrange apples for cheese filling.

8. Bake for about 10 minutes.

9. Reduce now the oven temperature to about 400 degrees and cook for another 25-30 minutes till firm as well as the apples are softened.

36. Salmons and Asparagus

|Calories: 258 kcal |Total time: 23min | Servings: 4 | Difficulty: Easy

Ingredients

* Wild-caught salmon, 16 oz

* Mayonnaise, 2 tablespoons, sugar-free

* Dijon mustard, 1 teaspoon

* Grated parmesan cheese, ¼ c

* Olive oil, 1 tablespoon

* Asparagus, 1 lb., fresh and ends trimmed

* Kosher salt, ½ teaspoon

* Black pepper, ¼ teaspoon, ground

- Lemons, 2

- Parsley, 2 tablespoons, chopped

Instructions

1. At 325 ° F, pre-heat the oven.

2. Rinse the salmon fillets and pat dry.

3. Lightly brush your finger through the filets and extract any bones.

4. In a small bowl, add the mayonnaise and Dijon mustard and blend.

5. Apply the mixture of mayonnaise over the salmon shell.

6. Sprinkle the cheese with parmesan over the top of the coated fish and press gently to secure.

7. Place the asparagus on the sheet saucepan and drizzle with the oil.

8. Toss the asparagus in the oil with tongs or your hands.

9. Lay the asparagus over the pan & leave room for salmon in the middle.

10. Place the salmon into the plate, CHEESE SIDE UP.

11. Split the lemons in half and put them somewhere on the sheet pan, split side up.

12. Sprinkle with salt and pepper over the whole shebang.

13. Bake for 18 minutes (for entire filet) or 12-15 minutes (for 4-ounce portions). Until 145 ° is read on a thermometer to the thickest section of the filet.

14. Remove from the oven & squeeze over the asparagus and salmon the required volume of juice from the lemons-extracting any seeds.

15. Garnish with parsley and eat warm or cold.

16. Grilled salmon with horseradish Sauce

37. Salmon Fillets

|Calories: 300 kcal |Total time: 25min | Servings: 4 | Difficulty: Easy

Ingredients

- The skin on or skinless salmon fillets, 4 – 6, 6 oz

- Olive oil, for coating salmon and grill

- Salt and freshly ground black pepper, as per taste

- Cream cheese, cubed into small cubes 4 oz

- Milk, ¼ c

- Homemade or store-bought horseradish sauce, plus more for serving, 3 tablespoons

Instructions

1. Pre-heat a grill to around 425 degrees F over medium-high heat. Brush with olive oil on both sides of the salmon (about 1 Tablespoon total), and season with salt and pepper on both sides.

2. Brush grill grates with oil & grill salmon for around 3 minutes per side or desired doneness.

3. Heat the cream cheese with milk in a saucepan over medium heat. The salmon is grilling, stirring until melted, around 1-2 min. Stir in horseradish and remove from heat.

4. Serve warm salmon with a creamy sauce flavored with horseradish.

Chapter 3: Kidney Friendly Renal Diet Dinner Recipes

1. Pesto-Crusted Catfish

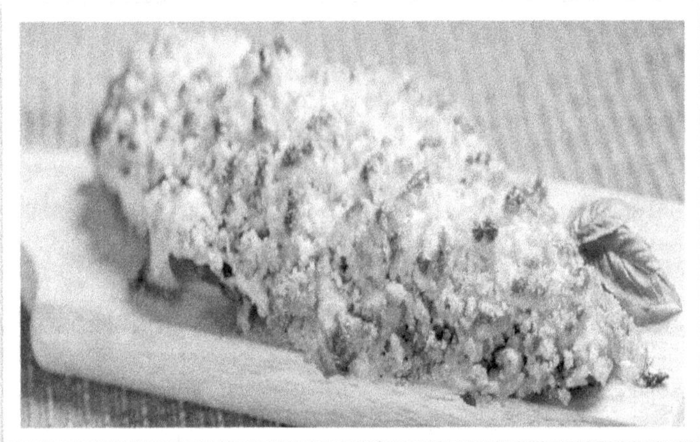

|Calories: 312Kcal |Total time: 45min | Servings: 6 | Difficulty: Easy

Ingredients

- Catfish 2 pounds (6 5-ounce pieces), filleted and boned

- Pesto, 4 teaspoons

- Panko breadcrumbs, ¾ cup

- Mozzarella cheese, ½ cup

- Olive oil, 2 tablespoons

Seasoning Blend (Chef McCargo's Signature)

- Garlic powder, 1 teaspoon

- Onion powder, 1 teaspoon

- Oregano ½ teaspoon, dried

- Red pepper flakes, ½ teaspoon

- Black pepper, ½ teaspoon

Instruction

1. Preheat oven to about 400° F.

2. Add all the seasonings inside a small bowl, mix and scatter even proportions on each side

of the fish.

3. Spread equal quantities of pesto (1 Teaspoon. each) over the fillets' top and set aside.

4. Take a medium bowl, then mix the bread, oil, and cheese crumbs and dredge the fish's pesto side till it is coated well.

5. Grease or spray the baking sheet generously with oil and put the fish pesto on the side of the tray, making space between the fillets.

6. Bake it at 400°Farenheit for about 15-20 minutes or till it becomes brown as per your desire on the bottom rack.

Let us Enjoy the Dinner

2. Smoking of Good Chicken (with Mustard Sauce)

|Calories:361cal |Total time: 15min | Servings: 6| Difficulty: Easy

Ingredients

- Chicken breast 2 pounds, finely diced (you may take boneless and skinless chicken breast minced thin)

- Shallots ¼ cup, cubed

- Scallions ¼ cup, fresh and chopped

- Flour, ½ cup

- Canola oil, ½ cup

- Chicken stock, 2 cups, low sodium

- Better Than Bouillon® Chicken Base 1 tablespoon, (low sodium)

- Brown mustard, 2 tablespoons

- Butter ½ stick, unsalted, chilled, and diced

  Seasonings:

- Black pepper, ½ teaspoon

- Italian seasoning, ½ teaspoon

- Parsley 1 tablespoon, dried

- Paprika 1 tablespoon, smoked

Instruction

1. In a small pan, add the pepper, the Italian spice, the paprika and the parsley, then mix them well.

2. Sprinkle a part of it on the breast piece of chicken and then add the rest to the flour.

3. Now heat the oil in a big sauté pan over medium-high flame.

4. Take 3 tablespoons of the flour and put it aside.

5. Dredge the chicken in the residual seasoned flour, then sauté for about 2-3 minutes per side.

6. Remove the chicken from the heat and then set aside on the counter to rest. Take all, but just a few tablespoons. Of the oil, then add the shallots with sauté until it becomes slightly translucent.

7. Mix in flour till it becomes smooth and steadily add stock while continuing to whisk. Now cook over medium-high heat for 5 minutes, then reduce the heat and mix it in the chicken bouillon, unsalted butter, and mustard.

8. Turn the heat off and add the chicken and juice sauce back to the pan, and mix. Plate and season with some scallions.

3. Meatloaf

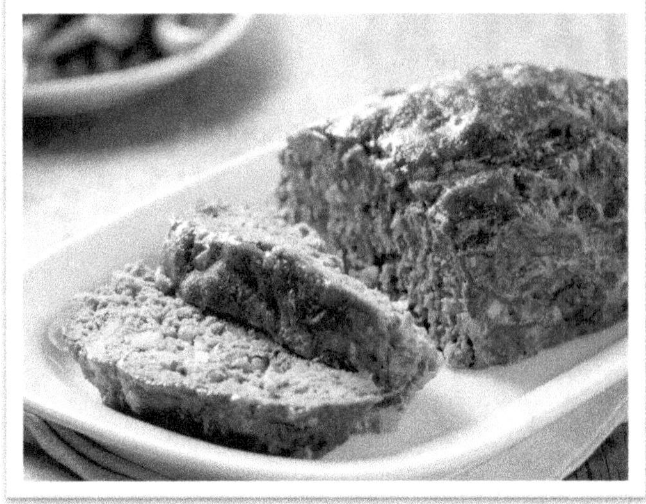

|Calories:367cal |Total time: 35min| Servings: 4| Difficulty: Easy

Ingredients

- Ground beef or crushed turkey, 1 pound, 85% lean

- Egg 1, beaten

- Panko breadcrumbs, ½ cup

- Mayonnaise, 2 tablespoons

Seasonings:

- Garlic powder, 1 teaspoon

- Onion powder, 1 teaspoon

- Better Than Bouillon® Beef Base 1 teaspoon (low sodium)

- Worcestershire sauce, 1 tablespoon, low sodium

- Red pepper flakes, ½ teaspoon

Instruction

1. Mix all the ingredients (other than the ground beef or the turkey) in a medium-sized bowl until well mixed. Now add the beef or turkey to the bowl and blend.

2. Pour the mixture into the meatloaf pan, or you may form it into an 8" x 4" elongated loaf or meatloaf form or form into 2 separate meatloaf forms and put it on the small baking sheet.

3. Cover it with the aluminum foil, then bake for about 20 minutes, then cut the foil and cook for another 5 minutes. Switch the oven and then let it settle in the oven for about 10 minutes before serving. Enjoy

4. Chicken and Gnocchi Dumplings

|Calories:362cal |Total time: 55min| Servings: 10| Difficulty: Easy

Ingredients

- Chicken breast, 2 pounds

- Gnocchi, 1 pound, store-bought

- Grapeseed or olive oil, ¼ cup

- Better Than Bouillon® Chicken Base 1 tablespoon, (low sodium)

- Chicken stock 6 cups, reduced sodium

- Celery ½ cup, fresh and finely cubed

- Onions ½ cup, fresh and finely cubed

- Carrots ½ cup, fresh and finely chopped

- Parsley ¼ cup fresh, chopped

- Black pepper, 1 teaspoon

- Italian seasoning, 1 teaspoon

Instruction

1. Put the stockpot on the burner, add the oil and set for a high flame.

2. Put the chicken in the hot oil and brown it from all sides till golden brown.

3. Add the celery, onions, and carrots, then cook them with the chicken till translucent. Now add chicken stock, then cook over high flame for about 20–30 minutes.

4. Reduce the heat and then add the chicken bouillon with the black pepper and the Italian seasoning, then mix. Add the gnocchi and cook it for about 15 minutes by stirring continuously.

5. Remove from the burner, garnish with the parsley, and serve.

5. Bourbon-Glazed Skirt Steak

|Calories:409cal |Total time: 45min| Servings: 6 | Difficulty: Easy

Ingredients

Bourbon Glaze:

- Shallots, ¼ cup diced

- Butter, 3 tablespoons, unsalted, cool, and diced

- Bourbon 1 cup

- Dark brown sugar, ¼ cup

- Dijon mustard, 2 tablespoons

- Black pepper, 1 tablespoon

Skirt Steak:

- Grapeseed oil, 2 tablespoons

- Oregano ½ teaspoon, dried

- Paprika ½ teaspoon, smoked

- Black pepper, 1 teaspoon

- Red wine vinegar, 1 tablespoon

- Skirt steak, 2 pounds

Instruction

Bourbon Glaze:

1. In a small frying pan over medium-high flame, brown the shallots in 1 Tablespoon of butter.

2. Reduce heat to a minimum, remove the saucepan from the burner, add bourbon, and put it again on the burner.

3. Cook it for about 10–15 minutes, or until around one third is reduced.

4. Now add the black pepper, the mustard and the brown sugar and mix until it becomes bubbly.

5. Switch off the heat and whisk in the residual 1 Teaspoon. Of cold, diced butter, stirring continuously until well mixed.

Steak Skirt:

1. Mix the first five ingredients in a gallon-sized sealed plastic container, add the steaks, and mix them well.

2. Enable steaks to marinate inside a container at room temperature for about 30-45 minutes.

3. Take the steaks out from the container, grill it for about 15-20 minutes on each side and then remove and let it stand for 10 minutes.

4. Cut and serve it with a dropping of sauce, or you may leave it whole and then brush with glaze and place it in the preheated broiler for about 4–6 minutes or until needed.

6. Chicken Pot Pie Stew

|Calories:388cal |Total time: 4hour| Servings:8 | Difficulty: Medium

Ingredients

- Chicken breast 1 ½ pound, "natural" fresh, boneless, and skinless

- Chicken stock 2 cups, reduced sodium

- Canola oil, ¼ cup

- Flour, ½ cup

- Carrots, ½ cup, fresh and chopped

- Onions ½ cup, fresh and chopped

- Celery ¼ cup, fresh and chopped

- Black pepper, ½ teaspoon

- Italian seasoning, 1 tablespoon, sodium-free (e.g., mccormick)

- Better Than Bouillon® Chicken Base 2 teaspoons (reduced sodium)

- Sweet peas ½ cup, fresh, frozen, and thawed

- Heavy cream, ½ cup

- Piecrust 1 frozen, cooked and broken into bite-size pieces

- Cheddar cheese, 1 cup low-fat

Instruction

1. Tenderize the chicken and sliced it into tiny cubes.

2. Put chicken and stock it in a wide saucepan and cook over medium-high flame for 30 minutes. In the meanwhile, mix the oil with flour till well mixed.

3. Then add slowly and whisk in a mixture of chicken broth until it is slightly thickened. Lower the heat to minimal or medium for 15 minutes.

4. Add broccoli, onions, celery, black pepper, Italian seasonings, and bouillon. Cook for another 15 minutes.

5. Switch off the flame, and now add the peas as well as the milk. Stir until well balanced.

Serve in mugs, then finish with fair quantities of cheese and for garnishing, use piecrust.

TIP: For quick cutting, freeze the breast piece of chicken for about thirty min, before cutting into pieces. Often put it in the fridge or freeze fresh meat or poultry instantly or within 2 hrs. of purchasing or preparation.

Alternative preparation of the crock-pot:

1. Put the crock-pot on full for about 4 hours.

2. Put oil, sauté carrots, onions, then celery for around 5 minutes before they are translucent.

3. Add flour and mix until the paste starts to shape, stirring continuously for around 3 minutes.

4. Add the chicken, the stock, the black pepper, the Italian seasoning, and the broth. Stir until well balanced.

5. Cover and let it simmer, mixing about once an hour. Approximately half hour before frying, add the cream with peas and mix. Cover and stir occasionally for about the last 30 minutes of preparation.

6. Cover with bits of piecrust and cheese. Enjoy

7. Baby Back Ribs BBQ (Sauce-less)

Calories: 324cal |Total time: 2.5hour| Servings: 12 | Difficulty: Easy

Ingredients

- Baby back ribs (about 3½ pounds), 2 slabs

- Fresh or frozen on the cob ears corn, 12 mini-

- Rub,1 portion

- Chef McCargo's (BBQ spice) rub

- Dark brown sugar 1 cup packed

- Black pepper, 1 teaspoon

- Red pepper flakes, 1 teaspoon

- Smoked paprika, 1 teaspoon

- Granulated garlic, 2 teaspoons

- Onion flakes dehydrated, 2 teaspoons

- Dark chili powder, 2 teaspoons

Instruction

1. Preheat an oven to 400 ° Fahrenheit

2. Rub the ribs from both sides with a blend.

3. Place the ribs on the rack-lined wire tray. Cover securely with aluminum foil and bake it for 1½ to 2 hours.

4. Take out from the oven, then remove the foil. Use tongs to put back the ribs. Drain any liquids out of the pan, then put the ribs again on the plate.

5. Cook for another 10-15 minutes or until crisp.

6. Let stay for 8-10 minutes, finally cut, and serve.

8. Spaghetti and Asparagus Carbonara

|Calories:304 |Total time: 10min| Servings: 6| Difficulty: Easy

Ingredients

- canola oil, 2 teaspoons

- fresh diced onions, 1 cup

- beaten egg, 1 large

- heavy cream, 1 cup

- chicken stock, ¼ cup

- spiral noodle pasta, 3 cups cooked,

- chopped fresh asparagus, 2 cups (about 1-inch-long pieces)

- black pepper freshly cracked coarse 1 teaspoon

- chopped fresh scallions, ½ cup

- bacon bits 3 tablespoons (meatless)

- Parmesan cheese shredded, 3 tablespoons

Instruction

1. In a broad non-stick saucepan, heat some oil over medium heat and sauté your onions until finely browned.

2. In the meantime, mix the egg with milk in a medium bowl until completely combined.

3. Now turn the heat down to medium and apply the creamy mixture to the onions. While stirring continuously with a wooden spoon, keep strolling until it begins to thicken. Around 4–6 minutes are required.

4. Add all the stock, the spaghetti, asparagus with the black pepper in a saucepan and stir for another 4-5 minutes or until the mixture is heated and well cooked.

5. Now lower the heat and place the carbonara in a serving bowl. Cover with scallions, bacon or cheese and serve hot.

9. Sweet Pepper Medley with Cabbage and Onion

|Calories:70cal |Total time: 30min| Servings: 4| Difficulty: Easy

Ingredients

- Red fresh bell pepper, ½ cup

- Green fresh bell pepper, ½ cup

- Yellow fresh bell pepper, ½ cup

- Freshly chopped onions, ½ cup

- Fresh shredded cabbage, 2 cups

- White vinegar, 3 tablespoons

- Canola oil, 1 tablespoon

- Brown sugar, 1 ½ teaspoons

- Dijon mustard, 1 ½ teaspoons

- Pepper, 1 ½ teaspoons

Instruction

1. Cut the bell peppers and make thin slices of 2-inch-long.

2. In a broad non-stick pan, mix bell peppers with onion and cabbage, then stir gently.

3. Combine the vinegar with the remaining ingredients in the pot, cover them tightly and shake vigorously.

4. Add the mixture of vegetables while stirring gently.

5. Sautee those over medium heat for few minutes or until the cabbage becomes soft.

10. Adobo-Marinated Tilapia Tapas

|Calories:254cal |Total time: 50min | Servings: 12 |Difficulty: Easy

Ingredients

- Tilapia filets piece, 6 3-ounce

- Wonton wrappers small, 48

- Non-stick cooking spray

Adobo Sauce:

- Spanish paprika, 3 tablespoons

- Oregano, 1 tablespoon

- Fresh chopped cilantro, 3 tablespoons

- Black pepper, 1 teaspoon

- Red pepper flakes, 1 teaspoon

- Wine vinegar red, ½ cup

- Extra-virgin olive oil, ¼ cup

Slaw Mix:

- Mayonnaise, ½ cup

- Chopped fresh garlic, 1 tablespoon

- Sliced thin fresh green scallions, ¼ cup,

- Rough cut fresh cilantro leaves, ¼ cup

- (shredded slaw mix) fresh cabbage, 4 cups

- Lemon juice ¼ cup

Instruction

1. Preheat your oven to 400 °.

2. Mix well the adobo ingredients continue mixing until fully combined and put aside.

3. Marinate the fillets of fish in a half cup of adobe sauce. Marination required 30 minutes.

4. Lightly spray on the baking sheet some non-stick spray and bake the fish for around 15 minutes at 400°, turning halfway through. Remove the mixture from the oven and put it aside.

5. Mix the leftover adobo sauce with garlic, the scallions and the cilantro using a medium bowl until fully combined. Add the cabbage and stir softly.

6. Spray a shallow muffin tin with a cooking spray. Set up the cups using a Winton wrapper.

7. Bake at 350 degrees F for 5 minutes, let them cool and pick out crispy wontons from the oven.

8. Place equal parts of the fish (cut or split into 48 pieces) directly on the wontons and cover equal quantities of the slaw mixture. Garnish with some cilantro leaves.

11. Crunchy and Sweet Coleslaw

|Calories:244cal |Total time: 10min | Servings:4 | Difficulty: Easy

Ingredients

- Shredded cabbage, 6 cups

- Chopped sweet onion, ½ cup

- Sugar, 1 cup

- Canola oil, 1 cup

- Celery seed, 1 teaspoon

- Rice vinegar, ½ cup

- yellow prepared mustard, 1 teaspoon

Instruction

1. Mix the chopped cabbage with the chopped onion in a big bowl.

2. In a mixer, mix all other items until well mixed.

3. Pour the dressing over cabbage and onion. Mix and refrigerate for a few minutes.

4. Serve it when chilled

12. Mediterranean Green Beans

|Calories:71cal |Total time: 6min | Servings: 4 | Difficulty: Easy

Ingredients

- Fresh green beans 1 pound, sliced into, 1-2" pieces

- Water, ¾ cup

- Olive oil, 2 ½ teaspoons

- Fresh minced garlic cloves, 3

- Fresh lemon juice, 3 tablespoons

- Ground black pepper, 1/8 teaspoon

Instruction

1. Get some boiling water in a broad non-stick skillet; then add the beans in this water, simmer for 3 minutes, and set aside after drain well.

2. Heat the skillet over medium heat and add some oil; with garlic and the beans, then Sautee them for 1 minute.

3. Add the juice and the pepper and further sauté for 1 minute.

4. Serve hot and enjoy.

13. Crunchy Lemon-Herbed Chicken

|Calories: 277cal |Total time: 45min | Servings: 4 | Difficulty: Easy

Ingredients

- Chicken tender, 2-ounce

- Chilled unsalted butter, 4 tablespoons

- Panko breadcrumbs, ½ cup

- Lemon juice, ¼ cup, plus 1 lemon zest

- Egg yolk 1

- Chopped fresh oregano, 1 tablespoon,

- Chopped fresh basil, 1 tablespoon

- Chopped fresh thyme, 1 tablespoon

- 3 tablespoons of water

Instruction

1. Heat 2 Tablespoon of butter over medium heat.

2. Add the zest of lemon and half number of herbs and breadcrumbs and leave the remaining ingredients to make a lemon sauce.

3. Beat the egg yolk.

4. Put chicken tenders in between two plastic wrap pieces, then beat it with a groove until it becomes weak but not torn. Dip the chicken in the mixture of eggs, then dip in a mixture of herbed breadcrumbs. Place them aside.

5. Heat 2 teaspoons of butter to medium heat.

6. Put the breaded chicken in the saucepan.

7. Cook chicken, around 2-3 minutes per side.

8. Remove the chicken and put it on the baking sheet for some time. Add the remaining herbs and the lemon juice to the same plate, then heat it until it simmers.

9. Turn off the heat; now add the remaining 2 teaspoons of butter into the sauce and whisk vigorously.

10. Cut the chicken.

11. Put the sliced chicken on the tray, pour the sauce all over the top for garnishing.

14. Chili Cornbread Casserole

|Calories:392 |Total time: 65min| Servings: 8| Difficulty: Easy

Ingredients

- Chili, 2

- Ground beef, 1 pound

- Diced onions, ½ cup

- Diced celery, ¼ cup

- Chopped jalapeño peppers, 2 tablespoons

- Chopped red or green peppers, ½ cup

- Chili powder, 1 tablespoon

- Granulated garlic powder, 1 tablespoon

- Dried onion flakes, 2 tablespoons

- Cumin, 1 tablespoon

- Ground black pepper, 1 teaspoon

- Tomato sauce½ cup, without added salt

- Water, ¼ cup

- French's® Worcestershire sauce, ¼ cup

- Kidney beans, 1 cup

- Shredded cheddar cheese, 1 cup

Cornbread:

- Cornmeal, ¼ cup

- Flour, ¾ cup

- Baking soda, ¼ teaspoon

- Cream of tartar, ½ teaspoon

- Sugar, ½ cup

- 1 beaten egg,

- Butter, 1 ½, tablespoons unsalted, melted

- Canola oil, ¼ cup

- Milk, ¾ cup

Instruction

1. Using a large saucepan, golden-brown ground beef and onions

    with celery, jalapenos, and bell peppers. Drain every excess of oil.

2. Add chili powder, onion, garlic, cumin, tomato sauce, black pepper, water, and the Worcestershire sauce with beans.

3. Cook for about 10 minutes.

4. Remove from heat, then dump in a 9" x 9" baking sheet, then spread the cheese over.

5. In a medium dish, add cornmeal, flour and baking soda with tartar cream and some sugar.

6. Beat the potato, melted butter, and oil, then add milk. Now combine the flour with egg mixture (if you have any good lumps, do not beat them). Pour the mixture with chili and bake it uncovered for 27-30 minutes, then cover and bake at 350°F for another 20 minutes, finally turn off oven leave to cool for 5 minutes.

15. Lemon Chicken Slow-Cooked

|Calories:197cal | Total time: 3hour| Servings: 4 | Difficulty: Easy

Ingredients

- Dried oregano, 1 teaspoon

- Ground black pepper, ¼ teaspoon

- Unsalted butter, 2 tablespoons

- Boneless chicken breast, 1 pound

- Low sodium chicken broth, ¼ cup

- Water, ¼ cup

- Lemon juice, 1 tablespoon

- Minced garlic cloves 2

- Chopped fresh basil, 1 teaspoon

Instruction

1. In a small container, combine the oregano with ground black pepper. Rubs these ingredients on the chicken.

2. Melt some butter in a medium-size saucepan over low heat.

3. Now cook and make the chicken brown in the melting butter and pass the chicken into a slow cooker.

4. Put chicken broth, sugar some lemon juice with the garlic in the saucepan.

5. Give it a boil so that browned parts get loosen in the skillet.

6. Pour it over the chicken.

7. Cover and adjust the slow cooker to medium flame for 2 1/2 hours.

8. Add basil to the chicken.

9. Cover, and again cook for another 15 minutes or until tender.

16. Green Bean Crunchy Casserole

|Calories:122cal |Total time: 25min | Servings: | Difficulty: Easy

Ingredients

- Green beans Fresh String, 12 oz

- Hot sauce, 2 tablespoons

- Gorgonzola, ¼ cup or cheddar cheese

- Unsalted and melted butter 2 tablespoons,

- Panko breadcrumbs, ½ cup

- Chopped green onions, 2 tablespoons

- Crushed unsalted tortilla chips, ½ cup

Instruction

1. Preheat an oven to 375 degrees F.

2. Chop the green beans to ~2" parts (heat for 6–8 minutes in a microwave-safe dish, damp with a wet paper towel)

3. Mix the sliced green beans and the hot sauce, then add this mixture to the saucepan.

4. Mix all the remaining ingredients in a cup. Spread the mixture uniformly over the string of green beans, then bake green bean (uncovered) inside the oven for 13–15 min. or until crisp.

17. Egg Noodles with Classic Beef Stroganoff

|Calories: 490cal |Total time: 25min | Servings: 6 | Difficulty: Easy

Ingredients

- Finely diced onions, 1 cup

- Beaten egg, 1

- French's® Worcestershire sauce, 2 tablespoons

- Breadcrumbs, ¼ cup

- Mayonnaise, 1 tablespoon

- Tomato sauce, 1 tablespoon without salt

- Ground beef, 1 pound

- Canola oil, 3 tablespoons

- Flour, 2 tablespoons

- Water, 3 cups

- Ground black pepper, 1 teaspoon

- (better then bouillon® beef) 4 teaspoons reduced sodium

- Sour cream, ¼ cup

- Chives, 2 tablespoons

- Cooked egg noodles, ½ package (12oz package),

- Unsalted butter, 2 tablespoons,

- Parsley, ¼ cup

- Chopped rosemary, 1 tablespoon

Instruction

1. Start by mixing the first 6 ingredients of the list and half the black pepper quantity in a big bowl.

2. Add beef and properly mix. Create 16 meatballs of the same scale.

3. In a wide saucepan over medium heat, start cooking stroganoff meatballs for few minutes or until browned.

4. Cook all the meatballs from all sides and pour some oil mixed with flour in the pan.

5. Add some water, mix the remaining black pepper, mix broth, and whisk until thickened for around 10 minutes.

6. Turn off the heat and whisk in the sour cream some chives, finely serve with egg noodles over it.

18. Roast Leg of Lamb (Herb-Crusted)

|Calories: 292kcal |Total time: 2hour| Servings: 4 | Difficulty: Easy

Ingredients

- Leg of lamb, 1 4-pound

- Lemon juice, 3 tablespoons

- Curry powder, 1 tablespoon

- Minced garlic, 2 cloves

- Ground black pepper, ½ teaspoon

- Sliced onions, 1 cup

- Dry vermouth ½ cup

Instruction

1. Preheat the oven to 400 degrees F.

2. Place the lamb leg on the roasting plate. Sprinkle 1 teaspoon of lemon juice.

3. Create a paste with 2Teaspoon. Of lemon juice, then add the remaining spices. Rub this paste on the lamb-leg.

4. Roast the lamb in a 400-degree oven for 30 minutes.

5. Drop the fat and add the vermouth and the onions.

6. Lower the heat to 325°F and roast for another 1 hour. Baste leg of the lamb. When the leg's internal temperature is 145°F, simply remove it from the oven and cool for about 2 minutes before serving.

19. Cilantro Slaw & Black Bean Burger

|Calories:380cal |Total time: 1hour| Servings: 6| Difficulty: Easy

Ingredients

- black beans, ½ cup rinsed

- Bulgur wheat, ½ cup

- Ground black pepper, 1 teaspoon

- Granulated garlic, 1 teaspoon

- Smoked paprika, ½ teaspoon

- French's® Worcestershire sauce 1 tablespoon,

- Onion flakes, 1 teaspoon

- Better than bouillon® beef, 1 tablespoon

- Onions, ½ cup

- Scallions, ¼ cup

- Flour, 2 tablespoons

- Slaw mix 3 cups (10-ounce bag) (also known as power blend)

- Balsamic vinegar, ¼ cup

- Cilantro, 2 tablespoons

- Sesame oil, 2 tablespoons

- Oil for searing*2 tablespoons canola

- Lime juice ¼ cup

- zest of, 1 lime

- Mayonnaise, ¼ cup

- Hamburger rolls, 6

Instruction

1. Preheat the oven to around 400 degrees F.

2. Mix black beans with bulgur wheat, add ground black pepper, mix it with spoon, add granulated garlic, some smoked paprika, and then add Worcestershire sauce and onion flakes 1 Teaspoon. Of water, then add beef bouillon and onions; finally, add 1⁄2 cup of scallions in a medium-sized dish.

3. Melt around 1⁄2 cup of the mixture in the burgers and refrigerate it until solid (not frozen).

4. Create vinaigrette with a combination of vinegar, add one tablespoon of cilantro with sesame oil and the lime juice.

5. Add 2 teaspoons of vinaigrette into the slaw mixture in a small pot, blend gently, and put aside in the refrigerator.

6. In another little bowl, combine the mayonnaise with the vinaigrette's remaining 2 teaspoons and put it aside.

7. Dust the black bean burgers using some flour and extract any waste. Bake for about 14 minutes and turn burgers halfway round.

8. Toast the rolls and scatter the same volume of the can. Add black bean burgers and finish with around 1⁄4 cup (or desired quantity) of slaw.

20. Smoky Cheese Sauce with Shrimp Grit Cakes & Egg

|Calories:390cal |Total time: 1.5hour| Servings:6 | Difficulty: Easy

Ingredients

- Beaten eggs, 4

- Unsalted butter, 2 tablespoons

- Diced onions, ½ cup

- Bacon½-inch pieces, 4 slices

- Deveined and peeled shrimp 12 16/20 count,

- Old bay® seasoning ,1 teaspoon

- Chopped chives, ¼ cup

- Chicken stock without salt, ½ cup,

- "better than bouillon" ® 2 teaspoons chicken flavor,

- 1 cup milk

- Grits, ½ cup

- Canola oil, 2 tablespoons

- Ground black pepper, ½ teaspoon

- Smoked paprika, ½ teaspoon

- Shredded cheddar cheese, ¼ cup

- Havarti, ¼ cup

- Canola oil, ¼ cup

- Flour, 3 tablespoons

Instruction

1. Heat the canola oil in a broad non-stick sauté pan, then scramble the eggs until cooked, not be too dry.

2. Place aside in the medium dish. Add the butter to the pan, then sauté the onions with shrimp, Old Bay®, then simply add about half of the chips until shrimps are slightly yellow.

3. Add chicken broth, eggs, and grits with bouillon and cook until finished according to box

instructions.

4. Turn off the heat and fold the egg, the bacon, and the shrimp mixture in the bowl. Place the mixture in lightly oiled baking dish 9" x 9" size and spread it until even coating is achieved, then cover and refrigerate it until solid.

5. Take the pan and break it into 6 squares.

6. Use a saucepan and heat the milk until it becomes hot. Now whisk in the cheese, the ground black pepper, some paprika and all the remaining chips until melted.

7. Place the sauce aside.

8. Heat half of the canola oil in a wide saucepan.

9. Lightly dust the grated cakes with flour and sauté them until they get golden brown.

10. Plate with equivalent quantities of smoked cheese sauce at the end

21. Bavarian Pot Roast Slow-Cooked

|Calories:313cal |Total time: 8.5hour| Servings: 12| Difficulty: Medium

Ingredients

- Beef chuck roast, 3 pounds

- Vegetable oil, 1 teaspoon

- Fresh ground ginger, ½ teaspoon

- Pepper, ½ teaspoon

- Whole cloves, 3

- Sliced apples, 2 cups

- Sliced onions, ½ cup

- Apple juice, ½ cup

- Flour, 4 tablespoons

- Water, 4 tablespoons

- Fresh apple slices for garnish

Instruction

1. Strip the beef roast from the extra fat.

2. Rinse and drain the pat. Rub some oil over the roast's top, now brush with ginger & pepper, then add the entire cloves.

3. Caramelize the pot roast using a hot oil pan on both sides.

4. Put the apples and the onions in a crock-pot.

5. Add the pot roast to and spill the apple juice all over the whole roast.

6. Cover and cook at low heat for 2 hours or maybe more depending upon the situation

7. Remove the roast from the slow cooker. Put it away but hold it warm. Strain the casserole juices and place them into the slow cooker again.

8. Switch the heat up to medium and thicken the liquid.

9. Create a smooth paste using flour and water, add to cooker.

10. Cover and boil until the mixture is thickened. Just before dinner, spill over the roast.

22. Spicy Beef Stir-Fry

|Calories:261cal |Total time: 25min| Servings: 4| Difficulty: Easy

Ingredients

- Separated cornstarch, 2 Tablespoons

- Sesame oil, ¼ teaspoon

- Sugar, ½ teaspoon

- Water, 2 tablespoons

- Large egg, 1

- Canola oil, 3 tablespoons

- Sliced beef round tip, 12 ounces

- Sliced green bell pepper, 1

- Sliced onions, 1 cup

- Ground chili pepper red, ¼ teaspoon

- Sherry, 1 tablespoon

- Soy sauce, 2 teaspoons

- Parsley as per need

Instruction

1. In a big bowl, whisk about 1 tablespoon of cornstarch, 1 & half tablespoon of water, 1 large egg size, 1 tablespoon of canola oil, and the beef. Now marinate for about 20 minutes.

2. In a separate cup, mix the leftover cornstarch with the water. Set it aside.

3. Heat 2 teaspoons of canola oil and add all the mixture to it (use a small saucepan for this). Cook it until the meat starts to brown.

4. Add orange bell pepper and the onion with some chili pepper. Finally, add the sherry. Cook about one minute. Add soya sauce, sugar, and some sesame oil.

23. Zesty Orange Tilapia

|Calories:133cal |Total time: 25min | Servings: 4 | Difficulty: Easy

Ingredients

- Tilapia, 16 ounces

- Julienned carrots, 1 cup

- Julienned celery, ¾ cup

- Sliced green onions, ½ cup

- Grated orange peel, 2 teaspoons

- Orange juice, 4 teaspoons

- Ground black pepper, 1 teaspoon

Instruction

1. Preheat the oven to 450 degrees F.

2. Mix broccoli, green onions with celery, and zest of the orange in a small bowl.

3. Break the tilapia into four equal parts.

4. Tear off four-wide squares of a foil and coat the foil with non-stick spray.

5. On each sheet of foil, put 1⁄4 of vegetables slightly off the middle and then top with the fish.

6. Now Sprinkle 1 Teaspoon of orange juice over each top. Season with some black pepper.

7. Fold the foil around the sides to create an envelope and put the foil right on the baking sheet.

8. Bake for around 10 minutes.   When finished, fish can split quickly with a fork.

9. Remove the bags and put them directly on plates.

10. Be alert when you open because of the steam.

24. Mashed Carrots with Ginger

|Calories:30cal | Total time: 15min | Servings: 3| Difficulty: Easy

Ingredients

- Baby carrots, 2 cups

- Chopped fresh ginger, ½ teaspoon

- Honey, ½ teaspoon

- Black pepper, ½ teaspoon

- Vanilla extract, ½ teaspoon

- Optional for garnish: fresh chives, 1 tablespoon.

Instruction

1. Boil or steam the carrots at high flame until the carrots are soft.

2. Drop heat to medium and mash all the carrots with the masher.

3. Add the remaining ingredients, i.e. (honey, ginger, vanilla extract with pepper), then mix until well combined.

25. Aromatic Herbed Rice

|Calories: 134cal |Total time: 5min| Servings:6| Difficulty: Easy

Ingredients

- Olive oil, 2 tablespoons

- Rice 3 cups, cooked (do not overcook)

- Garlic 4–5 cloves, fresh and sliced thin

- Cilantro 2 tablespoons, fresh and sliced

- Oregano 2 tablespoons, fresh and sliced

- Chives 2 tablespoons, fresh and sliced

- Red pepper flakes, ½ teaspoon

- Red wine vinegar, 1 teaspoon

Instruction

1. In a wide saucepan, heat the olive oil over a medium-high flame and sauté the garlic gently. Add now rice, herbs, and red pepper flakes, then simmer for about 2–4 minutes or until well blended.

2. Turn the heat off, add the vinegar, blend well and serve.

3. Chicken and Dumplings

26. Easy chicken on a slow cooker

|Calories:401cal |Total time:20min | Servings:6 | Difficulty: Easy

Ingredients

- Chicken 1 whole or chicken 3 lbs., sliced

- Water 2 cups of chicken broth low sodium

- Celery with leaves 1 stalk, cut fine

- Carrots 2-3, sliced

- Black pepper, 1/2 teaspoon

- Mace or nutmeg, 1/2 teaspoon

- Flour, 1/4 cup

- Eggs, 2

- Milk, 2/3 cup

- Baking powder, 3 teaspoons

- Flour, 2 cups

- Butter or margarine, 2 tablespoons, unsalted

Instruction

1. Take a slow cooker, then put the chicken, the vegetables, spices, and water inside it.

2. Add more water, sufficient to cover the chicken with around 1.

3. Switch the cooker on low flame for around 6-8 hours.

4. Take the chicken out from the ovenproof bowl.

5. Remove bones from meat. If you like, they may just slip off.

6. Cover and hold it wet.

7. Turn the slow cooker to increased heat. Add 1/4 cup of flour and whisk rapidly to prevent lumps.

8. Slice the butter with a knife and put it in two cups of flour.

9. Mix in wet ingredients for a firm dough and add the spoonful of it to the boiling broth.

10. Cover the cooker, lower the heat to stop boiling, then cook for about 15 minutes without uncovering it.

11. Place chicken in a wide serving plate and pour over the thickened sauce. Now serve it with dumplings.

27. Kidney Friendly Vegetable Soup

|Calories: 42Kcal |Total time: 50min| Servings:5| Difficulty: Easy

Ingredients

- Onion 1 medium, (150g / 6oz)

- Carrots 6 large, (6 x 140g / 5 ½ oz)

- Turnip 1 medium, (110g / 4 ½ oz)

- Celery 2 sticks, (60g / 2oz)

- Garlic 2 large cloves

- Chicken or vegetable low stock dices 1, a very little salt

- Bay leaf, 1

- Thyme, 1 teaspoon, fresh and sliced

- Black pepper, ¼ teaspoon

- Olive oil, 1 tablespoon

- Water 1 – 1.2 L

Instruction

1. Peel the onion, the carrot, and the turnip, then finely chop (for this, a food processor can accelerate the chopping process)

2. Dice the garlic and the celery finely.

3. Put the thinly sliced carrot, turnip inside a big pot, and then add water of about 4 times of their volume. Bring it to boil and cook until tender.

4. During when carrot and the turnip are frying, flame the olive oil in the frying pan.

5. Now add the onion, garlic, and celery once the oil is quietly hot. Put the vegetables in oil with a spoon to coat them.

6. Cover the pan with the lid and leave for half-fry over a low flame until softened. It is going to take around 15 minutes.

7. Shake or open the pot from about time to time, then mix to make sure it is burning or stuck.

8. Add the boiling carrot with turnip and blend.

9. Making chicken or vegetable stock via adding one very low salted vegetable or as per choice chicken stock cube into 1-1,2 Liter of boiling water.

10. Put the stock in the mixture of vegetables

11. Add now the bay leaf to the thyme

12. Season with some pepper

13. Put to a boil, after this cook for thirty min (or until the vegetables are cooked) without covering with a lid.

14. Drop the leaf of the Bay. Mix the broth until creamy by using a food processor.

15. Extra water may be applied to getting a thin soup.

28. Tuna Dip

Calories:700cal|Total time: 20min| Servings: 8 | Difficulty: Easy

Ingredients

- Cream cheese 250g, softened

- Onion 2 Tablespoon, finely sliced

- Garlic 1/2 clove, crushed

- Horseradish, 1 Tablespoon., prepared

- Worcestershire sauce pepper 1 Teaspoon.

- Sour cream, 1/2 cup

- Tuna 100g can be drained and scaled

Instruction

1. Mix cheese, tomato, garlic, horseradish, etc.

2. Worcestershire sauce and some chili.

3. Blend with the sour cream.

4. Attach the tuna and combine thoroughly.

29. Pumpkin Strudel

Calories: 180cal |Total time: 30min| Servings: 8 | Difficulty: Easy

Ingredients

- Canned pumpkin 11/2 cups, sodium-free, not the sweet one

- Nutmeg, 1/8 teaspoon, grated

- Vanilla extract, 1 teaspoon, pure

- Sugar, 4 tablespoons, divided

- Cinnamon, 11/2 teaspoons, ground and divided

- Butter 1/2 stick (4 tablespoons), without salt and melted

- Phyllo dough 12 sheets, (if frozen then follow directions for defrosting on the package)

Instruction

1. Place the oven rack inside the center of the oven. Now preheat the oven to about 375 degrees Fahrenheit.

2. In a medium cup, add the nutmeg with canned pumpkin, two tablespoons of sugar, vanilla extract, and 1/2 Teaspoon. Of cinnamon till well combined.

3. Use a pastry brush, cover the bottom of a medium-sized non-stick sheet pan with a tiny portion of melted butter.

4. Place a single layer of phyllo dough onto a tidy work surface and spray with some butter. Build a pile of phyllo sheets coated with butter in such a way that every other phyllo sheet is coated with butter. Note: Hold the leftover phyllo dough sheets wrapped with plastic cover until ready to use i.e., prevent them from drying out. Be sure to save some melted butter from coating the rolled filled strudel from the top.

5. When all 12 sheets have been used, pour the mixture uniformly over one of the stack's large side. Now start rolling from the loaded end to the unloaded end, make sure the seam end faces down.

6. Move the roll to the greased tray's seam side, then brush it with the remaining butter.

7. After this, mix the remaining two tablespoons. Of sugar and one teaspoon. Of cinnamon in a shallow cup. Spray over the top as well as the sides of the strudel.

8. Bake in the center rack until it becomes golden brown, around 12–15 minutes.

9. Take the tray out from the oven and enable toasted strudel to stand for about 5–10 minutes to make the core to settle before cutting. Using a small knife to break the roll into eight bits. Serve it.

30. BBQ Asparagus

|Calories:86cal |Total time: 20min| Servings: 6 | Difficulty: Easy

Ingredients

- Asparagus, 1/2 lb., fresh (12 – 15 large spears)
- Extra-virgin olive oil, 2-3 Tablespoon.
- Pepper, 1/2 Teaspoon.
- Lemon juice, 2-3 Tablespoon.

Instruction

1. Add oil, lemon juice, and black pepper in a shallow dish large enough to roll the asparagus and cover the mixture almost completely. Now mix them well.
2. Clean and cut the woody ends of asparagus spears. Tip: Keep the asparagus spear just under the tip from one side and at the top from the other and mix gently. Normally, the spear will offer at which woody ends stop, and the soft asparagus will begin.
3. Roll the asparagus inside a bowl with a mixture of oil and leave for some time. Put the tray onto the bowl to prevent the oil from leaking, keep it in the refrigerator for marination before the grill becomes ready.
4. Prepare for charcoal or gas barbecue, then heat it at medium-high flame.
5. Gently spray vegetable grilling tray or a grill bucket or maybe a sheet made of heavy-duty tin, folded in a deep olive oil spraying tray to prevent the spears from binding the plate.
6. Arrange the asparagus on a vegetable grilling plate and spill any leftover oil from the bowl onto the spears.
7. Grill the asparagus onto the tin foil or in the pan until tender and brown, regularly rotating for around 5 minutes. Now transfer to the tray. Serve hot or as per your choice at room temperature.

31. Kidney friendly Salad of Green beans

|Calories: 232 kcal |Total time: 27min| Servings: 6| Difficulty: Easy

Ingredients:

- Green beans fresh, 1 lb.
- Palm hearts, 2 cups, sliced

- Black olives, 3/4 cup, cut in half and drained

- Bell pepper red 1 cup, cubed and roasted

- Feta cheese, 1/2 cup, crumbled

- Black pepper, freshly ground

Dressing ingredients:

- Balsamic vinegar 1 tablespoon

- Lemon juice 2 tablespoons, fresh-squeezed

- Olive oil 1/3 cup

- Lemon zest 1 teaspoon.

- Fresh oregano 2 tablespoons, sliced

- Basil 2 tablespoon, fresh and sliced

Instructions

1. Trim green beans end.

2. Cut the beans into about 2" long pieces.

3. Steam beans in a big pot having a lid tight-fitting or a vegetable steamer (electric), using a steamer insert until they are some tender-crisp.

4. When beans are tender as you would like them, take off the steamer and immediately plunge into an ice water bowl to halt the cooking.

5. Remove the beans to a colander and allow them to drain and cool for about 15 mins, then spread the beans on towels on paper and then blot dry.

6. While the beans cook, slice, and drain the palm hearts, drain & red peppers chop, drain and cut olives in half, then measure the feta.

7. Combine lemon juice, balsamic vinegar, olive oil, chopped oregano, lemon zest & chopped basil & process until the herbs are chopped very thinly. The dressing is well mixed.

8. Combine drained beans and sliced palm heart, olive halves, & red pepper chopped to assemble the salad.

9. To moisten salad, add dressing as required and gently combine.

10. Add the feta cheese & stir to make the feta barely mix.

11. Grind black pepper & serve straight away.

12. This can keep inside the refrigerator for several days but bring the leftovers to room temp before serving.

32. Cauliflower soup

|Calories: 577 kcal |Total time: 35min| Servings: 6 | Difficulty: Easy

Ingredients

- Vegan butter, 1/4 cup

- Onion, 1 large

- Garlic, 3 cloves

- Cauliflower, 1 large head

- Sprigs, 2

- Water, 5 cups

- Vegan cream, 1 cup

- Small lemon

Instructions

1. Prep: Proceed with the ginger and garlic first. Split the asparagus into florets. Since you can break that down while it heats, they will be on the broadside.

2. Sauté: Heat oil or water over medium heat in a heavy bottom pan, sauté the onion for 6 min, add the garlic and cook for another 1 minute.

3. Transfer remaining ingredients: mix in cauliflower, thyme, salt and pepper shake, and water/broth.

4. Simmer: Carry the chunky soup to a boil, cover, decrease heat and steam, stirring regularly, for 20 minutes.

5. Stir in the vegan dairy or plant milk & lemon juice, apply cream + lemon.

6. Puree: Until the soup has stopped, allow to cool for ten min. Puree the soup to optimal

strength, utilizing an induction processor or cup processor. Where appropriate, sprinkle with salt and pepper. Heat under low before it warms up as required.

7. Serve with a few allocated toasted bits of cauliflower, organic cream drizzle, or new crushed chili pepper. Add a dash of red pepper flakes or crushed bay leaves for a little spice. Mix with baked Organic Bread or Vegan Naan, smooth and chewy to soak up the juices.

8. Store: The leftovers can be kept in a sealed jar in the fridge for up to 6 days. Refrigerate for up to 2-3 months to keep longer.

33. Kidney friendly Cauliflower Rice

|Calories: 292 kcal |Total time: 60min | Servings: 4 | Difficulty: Easy

Ingredients

- Cauliflower, 1 head

- Neutral oil, 2 tablespoons

- Scallions, 1 bunch

- Garlic, 3 cloves

- Ginger, 1 tablespoon

- Carrots, 2

- Celery stalks, 2

- Red pepper, 1

- Vinegar, 2 tablespoons

- Soy sauce, 3 tablespoons

- Sriracha, 2 teaspoons

Directions

- Pulse cauliflower in a food processor tank until the mixture resembles starch, for 2 to 3 minutes. Place on aside.

- Heat the oil over moderate heat in a large pan. Apply the scallions, garlic & ginger, then stir-fry for around 1 minute, until fragrant.

- Connect the carrots, celery & red pepper, and stir-fry for 9 to 11 minutes, till the vegetables are soft.

- Stir cauliflower rice until it starts becoming white, 3 to 5 minutes more. Stir in the frozen peas and toss together well.

- Stir in the soy sauce, rice vinegar, then Sriracha, then throw together. Place on aside.

34. Chicken Parmesan

|Calories: 441 kcal |Total time: 28min | Servings: 2 | Difficulty: Easy

Ingredients

- Chicken, 8-ounce, boneless

- Egg, 1

- Whipping cream 1 tablespoon

- Beef rinds, 1 ½ ounce

- Parmesan cheese 1-ounce

- Salt, ½ teaspoon

- Garlic powder, ½ teaspoon

- Red pepper flakes, ½ teaspoon

- Black pepper ½ teaspoon, ground

- Italian seasoning, ½ teaspoon

- Tomato sauce, ½ cup

- Mozzarella cheese ¼ cup

- Ghee, 1 tablespoon

Instructions

Place the oven rack from the heat source about six inches, then heat the broiler for the oven.

Slice the chicken breast sideways from one hand across the middle to about 1/2 inch from the other. Open both two sides and unfold as an open text. Quarter chicken smooth to around one and a half inches high.

Together mix egg & cream in a mug.

Combine broken rinds of pork, Parmesan cheese, mustard, powder of garlic, red flakes of pepper, black pepper, and Italian bowl seasoning; move breading to a pan.

Dip the chicken into a mixture of the eggs, cover entirely. Push the chicken onto breading; cover the two sides thickly.

Heat a squash over medium to high flame; add ghee. Put the chicken within the pan; cook until the center is no longer yellow, & the juices move clear, approximately 3 minutes per hand. A center-inserted thermometer of instant-read can register at least 165 degrees F. Be mindful of holding breading in position.

Place the chicken onto a baking dish. Tomato sauce on top; mozzarella cheese on top.

Boil for about 2 minutes, before the cheese is fizzing and lightly colored.

35. Chicken with olive oil

|Calories: 450 kcal |Total time: 28min | Servings: 2 | Difficulty: Easy

- Olive oil, 2 tablespoons

- Garlic cloves, 7

- Parsley, ½ cup, fresh

- Balsamic vinegar, 1 tablespoon

Instructions

1. To 225 ° C (450 ° F), preheat the oven.

2. Place the pieces of chicken in a baking pan grated with butter. Generous of salt & pepper.

3. Drizzle lemon juice and balsamic vinegar over the chicken bits and olive oil. Sprinkle parsley and garlic around it.

4. Bake the chicken for around 30–40 minutes, until garlic slices have changed color and roast. The baking period could be higher if the scale of the drumsticks is greater. Reduce the temperature a little at the top.

5. Serve.

Chapter 4: Kidney Friendly Renal Diet Dessert Recipes

1. Kidney friendly Syrup Sponge Pudding

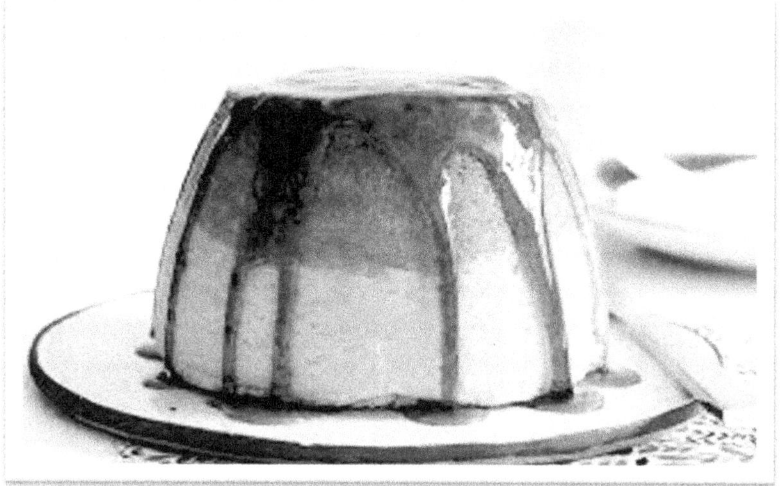

Calories: Kcal 546 |Total Time: 1 hour| Serves: 4| Difficulty: Easy

Ingredients

- Softened unsalted butter ,100g (3½oz)

- Caster sugar, 100g (3½oz)

- 2 eggs

- Self-rising flour, 100g (3½oz)

- Golden syrup, 6 tablespoons

Instructions

1. In a pan or food processor, put cream, butter and some sugar together.

2. Add one egg and combine it gently with flour. Insert the other egg and combine thoroughly and mix

3. Add mixture in a buttered bowl and spoon your cake mixture in it.

4. Bake for about 35-40 minutes at about 200 ° C (180 ° C fan)/400 ° F/Gas 6, unless a skewer originates out clean. Top with syrup.

5. Serve.

2. Kidney friendly rice Pudding

Calories: 365 kcal| Total time: 50 min |Serves: 6| Difficulty: medium

Ingredients

- Pudding rice, 200g (7oz)

- Soya milk (unsweetened), 800ml

- Sugar, 4 tablespoons

- Salt ½, teaspoon

- Vanilla extract, ½ teaspoon

- Cinnamon powder, ¼ teaspoon

- Nutmeg powder, ¼ teaspoon

Instructions

1. In a wide skillet, add soy milk & rice, then mix and boil on medium heat.

2. Reduce the heat after boiling and cook about 20 minutes or when the rice is quite tender.

3. Add butter, vanilla extract & salt, then roast, stirring regularly, for the next 2 minutes.

4. Load the rice pudding onto serving plates and, if appropriate, dust with cinnamon or nutmeg.

5. Serve instantly (warm) or cool down rice pudding and serve it cold.

3. Kidney friendly apple crumble

Calories: 608 kcal | Total time: 50 min |Serves: 4 |Difficulty: Easy

For the crumble

- Plain flour, 300g (10½oz) sieved

- A pinch of salt

- Sugar, 175g (6oz)

- Unsalted butter, 200g (7oz)

For the filling

- Apples, cut into ½ in pieces, 450g (1lb)

- Sugar, 50g (2oz)

- Plain flour, 1 tablespoon

- Ground cinnamon, 1 pinch

Instructions

1. Preheat an oven to about 180 degrees C (160 degrees Fan)/350 degrees F/Gas 4.

2. In a large bowl, put the sugar and flour and combine well. Mix the butter cubes into the flour mixture at the same moment. Gently rub until the combination is comparable to breadcrumbs.

3. Put the fruit and add sugar, starch and flour and cinnamon in a big bowl. Stir well and be cautious not to tear the fruit off.

4. Butter another 24 cm/9 sized ovenproof dish. Pour the mixture of fruits into it. Sprinkle the crumble mixture evenly,

5. Bake for 40-45 minutes in the oven till the crumble has browned and bubbling fruit blend.

6. Serve.

---

4. Renal friendly Lemon Cheesecake

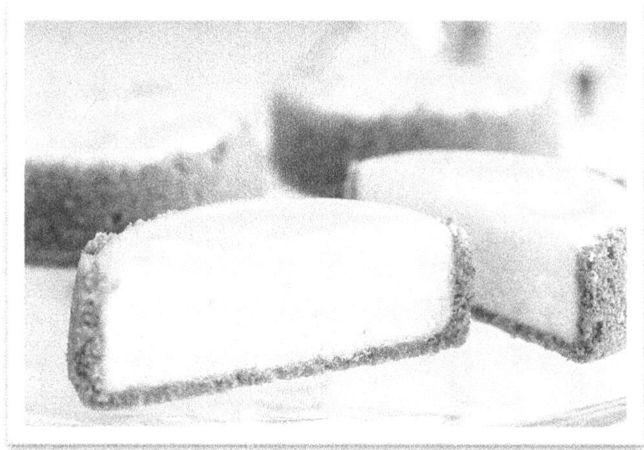

Calories: 4 hrs. 25 min |Total time: 6 hours |Serves: 6| Difficulty: High

Ingredients

For the base

- Digestive biscuits 200g (7oz)

- Soft unsalted butter 100g (3½oz)

- For the topping

- Cream cheese 1 packet

- Single cream 1 tub

- Icing sugar 250g (9oz)

- 1 lemon juice

Instructions

1. In a food processor, whizz the biscuits until you have perfect crumbs and then add butter via the nozzle in tiny bits while the butter is in tiny pieces.

2. Butter a tin, then push hard into the foundation mixture's bottom to set the tin, placed it in the fridge.

3. Mix the cream until enough thickened to almost retain its form

4. In the cream cheese package, beat till the mix is soft.

5. Insert sifted icing sugar, lemon juice, then beat before you can beat again the smooth, dense consistency is obtained.

6. Place the topping on the base and scatter it, bring that tin back in the tin, refrigerate before the topping is set.

5. Renal friendly cherry shortbread

Calories: 188 kcal |Total time: 1 hour 20 min |Serves: 6| Difficulty: medium

Ingredients

- Unsalted butter, 125g (4oz)

- Caster sugar, 55g (2oz)

- Plain flour, 180g (6oz)

Instructions

1. Warm the oven to 190 ° C (170 ° C ventilator)/375 ° F/Gas 5.

2. Together, mix the sugar and butter once smooth.

3. To have a smooth paste, whisk in the flour.

4. Apply (if using the cherries and gently stir to blend.

5. Switch on to a working surface and roll out softly until the paste is done.

6. Break it into fingers or rounds and put it on a baking tray. Sprinkle with the sugar and cool for 20 minutes in the refrigerator.

7. Bake for 15-20 minutes in the oven or until golden-brown pale. Cool aside on a wire shelf.

6. Kidney friendly Victoria Sponge Cake

Calories: 558 kcal |total time:1 hour | Serves 10 |Difficulty: Easy

Ingredients

- Unsalted butter, 250g (9oz)

- Caster sugar, 250g (9oz)

- Eggs, 4 media

- Self-rising flour, 250g (9oz)

- Double cream, 50ml

- Raspberry jam, 5 tablespoons

Instructions

1. Grease two tins of 20 cm of shallow cake and then line with baking **paper.** Preheat the oven to 180 degrees C (160 degrees Fan)/350 degrees F/Gas 4.

2. In a wide bowl, put the softened butter and sugar and beat until very fluffy and pale.

3. Apply to the mixture an egg and a huge spoon of flour and beat again. Until all the eggs are incorporated, repeat this process.

4. If there is no falling consistency in the mixture (i.e., simple drops Remove from a spoon), apply a milk splash.

5. Divide between the two tins, smooth the surface, and bake in the mixture for 25 minutes in the microwave.

6. They can be sandwiched while the cakes are baked and cooled. Before soft peaks shape, whisk the double cream. Jam spreading either of the cakes on the ground and then layer the whipped cream on the top.

7. Decorate and serve.

7. Easy Flapjacks

Calories: 108 kcal| Total time: 40 mins| serves :4 |Difficulty: easy

Ingredients

- Porridge oats, 250g (9oz)

- Melted unsalted butter, 125g (4oz)

- Brown sugar, 25g (4oz)

- Golden syrup, 2-3 tablespoons

Instructions

1. In a food processor or large tub, put all the ingredients and Combine, make sure that the oats maintain their texture

2. Grease a baking tin loosely in all the mixture with butter and spoon.

3. Push the back of the spoon onto the corners such that the paste is smooth. And the combination is scored into 12 squares.

4. Put in the oven and bake until golden brown, at 180 °C (160 °C fans)/350 °F/Gas.

8. Madeira Cake

Calories: 397 kcal | Total time: 1 hr. 30 mins| Serves 6-8 |Difficulty: Easy

Ingredients

- Unsalted butter, 175g (6oz) at room temperature

- Caster sugar, 175g (6oz)

- 3 eggs

- Self-rising flour, 250g (9oz)

- Milk, 2-3 tablespoon

- 1 lemon

Instructions

1. Preheat the oven around 180 degrees C (160 degrees Fan)/350 degrees F/Gas 4.

2. Grease a circular cake tin of 18cm/7in, cover the foundation with greaseproof Paper and paper oil.

3. In a cup, cream your butter & sugar together until they are pale & fluffy.

4. Beat the chickens, one at a time and beat the combination in them well. Each one and applies the last egg to a tablespoon of flour. Prevent the curdling of the mixture.

5. Mix the flour and fold it softly with sufficient milk to create a mixture. It comes out of the spoon steadily. Fold the lemon zest in it.

6. Spoon the blend into the packed tin and level the surface slightly. Bake and bake for 30-40 minutes on the middle shelf of the oven, or until golden-brown on top and a skewer inserted in the center comes out clean.

9. Spelt Waffle

Calories: 222 kcal| Total time: 25 mins| Serving: 4| Difficulty: Easy

Ingredients

- Spelt Flour, 1 cup

- Sea Moss, 1 teaspoon.

- Hemp Milk, ¼ cup

- Sea Salt, a pinch

- Allspice Powder, ½ teaspoon.

Instructions

1. To start with, whisk the oil on the waffle maker. Now preheat the waffle maker swiftly. Next, dump the dough into the maker. Lastly, cook the waffles around five to six mins over medium flame or until browned. Only serve it warm.

10. Kidney friendly blueberry cake

Calories: 222 kcal| Total time: 55 mins |Serving: 6 |Difficulty: Easy

Ingredients

- Chickpea Flour, 1 cup

- Blueberries, 1 cup

- Spelt Flour, 2/3 cup + 1 tablespoon.

- Sea Salt a pinch

- Water, ¾ cup

- Grapeseed Oil, 2 tablespoons

- Agave Nectar, 6 tablespoons.

Instructions

1. First, put all the ingredients you need to cook in a blender, then blend for three minutes until there are no more chunks in it. Next, move the paste to a parchment baking pan, which must be properly paper-lined and distribute it uniformly. Bake for about twenty-eight to thirty minutes or when golden browned and baked. Enjoy

11. Banana Nut Muffins

Calories: 222 kcal| Total time: 50 mins| Serving: 12| Difficulty: Easy

Ingredients:

- Spelt Flour, 3 ½ cup

- Bananas 3, mash them

- Spring Water, as desired

- Walnuts, 1 cup, sliced

- Salt a Pinch

- Date Syrup, 1 tablespoon.

- Perrier, ¾ cup

Instructions

1. To make this wonderful cake, add the mashed banana and the date syrup in the bowl and mix it until well. Mix in spelled flour, then add salt and mix until combined.

2. Mix it again. And mix the Perrier and the walnuts. Stir it well. If the batter appears to be too dense, add a little water as required. Now add the mixture into the molds of the muffin and line them with 3/4. Lastly, bake at 350 p.m. for about eighteen to twenty minutes or till it is bake.

12. Kidney friendly blueberry Spelt Pancakes

Calories: 190 kcal| Total time: 20 mins| Serving: 2| Difficulty: Easy

Ingredients

- Spelt Flour, 2 cups

- Sea Moss, ¼ teaspoon.

- Hemp Milk, 1 cup

- Agave Syrup, ½ cup

- Spring Water, ½ cup

- Blueberries, ½ cup

- Grapeseed oil 2 tablespoon.

Instructions

1. For this balanced breakfast dish, add the spelled flour, the agave syrup, the sea moss, and the grapeseed oil uniformly in a big mixing pot. Now, slowly pour the hemp milk into it and the water into it. Then gently press in the blueberries.

2. After that, heat a broad pan over medium-high flame. Once the pan is hot, spray it with oil. Then, add a spoon full of the mixture and cook every side for about 3 to 5 minutes.

3. Now finally, serve them hot.

13. Strawberry Sorbet

Calories: 22 kcal| Total time: 4 hr.| Serving: 3| Difficulty: Easy

Ingredients

- Date Sugar, ½ cup

- Strawberries, 2 cups

- Spring Water, 2 cups

- Spelt Flour, 1 ½ teaspoon.

Instructions

1. Begin by combing date sugar, spelled flour, and spring water in a medium-sized pot. Next, heat the mixture over low heat and cook for 8 to 10 minutes or till thickened. After that, take off the pot from the heat and allow it to cool. Once cooled, puree the strawberries in a blender.

2. Now, mix the strawberry puree to the flour mixture and give everything a good stir. Then, pour the mixture into a container and keep it in the freezer. Cut the frozen sorbet to pieces and place it in the blender or food processor.

3. Blend until smooth and return the container to the refrigerator for a minimum of 4 hours.

4. Finally, serve the chilled strawberry sorbet.

14. Strawberry Ice Cream

Calories: 354 kcal| Total time: 20 mins| Serving: 3-4| Difficulty: Medium

Ingredients

- Hemp Milk, ¼ cup

- Frozen strawberries, 1 cup

- Agave Syrup, 1 tablespoon.

- Frozen Baby, Bananas, 5

- Ripe Avocado, ½ of 1

Instructions

1. Place all ingredients necessary to make this ice cream into a high-speed blender. Mix them for 2-3 minutes or till the mixture is smooth.

2. Check for sugar and, if appropriate, insert more agave syrup.

3. Finally, move to the freezer-friendly jar and freeze for 4-6 hours

15. Blueberry Muffins

Calories: 383 kcal| Total time: 14 mins| Serving: 12| Difficulty: Easy

Ingredients

- Two and a half cup, almond flour

- One-third cup, keto-friendly sugar

- One and a half teaspoon, baking powder

- Half teaspoon, baking soda

- Half teaspoon, kosher salt

- One-third cup, melted butter

- One-third cup, unsweetened almond milk

- Three large eggs

- One teaspoon, pure vanilla extract

- Two-third cup, blueberries

- Half lemon zests

Instructions

1. Start by preheating the oven to a temperature of 350 ° and put in a muffin tray with cupcake liners.

2. In a big container, stir together almond flour, Swerve, baking soda, baking powder, and salt. Gently stir in melted butter, eggs, and vanilla once mixed.

3. Gently fold the blueberries and the lemon zest until uniformly spread. Scoop equivalent quantities of the mixture into each liner of cupcakes and bake until softly golden. A toothpick inserted into the middle of the muffin comes out clean; this will happen within 23 minutes. Let it cool slightly before serving.

16. Gingersnap Baked Apples

Calories: 343 kcal| Total time: 1 hr.| Serving: 8| Difficulty: Easy

Ingredients

- Gingersnap cookies, 3 ounces

- Brown sugar, 2 tablespoons

- Apples, 4 sweet

- Butter rinsed, ¼ cup

- Whipping cream, ½ cup

Instructions

1. Gingersnaps and brown sugar whirl into small crumbs in the mixer or the food processor.

2. Cut around cores up to around 3/4 of the way through apples with a thin, sharp knife, beginning from stem ends; pick out cores with the spoon, creating a 1 1/2-inch-wide cavity and then keeping bases unaffected. - In the shallow 2 3-quart baking dish, set the apples moderately apart.

3. Spoon each cavity with 1 tablespoon of ginger snap mixture and finish with 1/2 tablespoon of butter. Sprinkle the apples generously with the remaining blend of ginger.

4. Bake in a standard or convection oven of 375o until apples are soft, around 45 minutes until pierced. Shift into individual bowls and, if necessary, pour 2 teaspoons of cream around each.

17. Apple cider donut bites

Calories: 164 kcal| Time: 30 mins| Serving 12 | Difficulty: easy

Ingredients

Donut bites:

- Almond flour, 2 cups

- Swerve sweetener, ½ cup

- Whey protein powder unflavored, ¼ cup

- Baking powder, 2 teaspoons

- Cinnamon, ½ teaspoon

- Salt, ½ teaspoon

- Large eggs, 2

- Cup water, 1/3

- Butter melted, ¼ cup.

- Apple cider vinegar, 1 ½ tablespoon

- Apple extract, 1 ½ teaspoon

Coating:

- Swerve sweetener, 1/4 cup

- Cinnamon, 1 to 2 teaspoons

- Butter melted, 1/4 cup.

Instructions

1. Oven Preheated to325f, then grease well a tiny muffin pan (use a standard muffin box with 24 cavities).

2. Mix all the almond meal, sweetener, powder of protein, dried powder, spices & salt in the large bowl. Whisk till it is mixed in milk, sugar, butter, cider vinegar & apple extract.

3. Divide the mixture between the wells of the prepared tiny muffin pan. Bake for 15-20 mins, till the cup's cakes, are hard to touch. Remove & allow it to cool for 10 mins, then Switch to the wire rack to completely cool.

4. Mix both sweetener & spices in a tiny bowl. Dip a full bite of donut in the softened butter, fully covering it. Then roll the combination into each donut snap.

18. Gingersnap Baked Apples

Calories: 346 kcal| Preparation time: 1 hr.| Servings: 8 | Difficulty: Easy

Ingredients

- Gingersnap cookies, 3 ounces

- Brown sugar, 2 tablespoons

- Apples, 4 sweet

- Butter rinsed, 1/4 cup

- Whipping cream, 1/2 cup

Instructions

1. Gingersnaps and brown sugar whirl into small crumbs in the mixer or the food processor.

2. Cut around cores up to around 3/4 of the way through apples with a thin, sharp knife, beginning from stem ends; pick out cores with the spoon, creating a 1 1/2-inch-wide cavity and then keeping bases unaffected. - In the shallow 2 3-quart baking dish, set the apples moderately apart.

3. Spoon each cavity with 1 tablespoon of ginger snap mixture and finish with 1/2 tablespoon of butter. Sprinkle the apples generously with the remaining blend of ginger.

4. Bake in a standard or convection oven of 375o until apples are soft, around 45 minutes until pierced. Shift into individual bowls and, if necessary, pour 2 teaspoons of cream around each.

19. Pear and Ginger Cake

Calories: 453 kcal| Preparation time: 45 mins| Servings: 4 | Difficulty: Medium

Ingredients

- Butter, ½ cup

- Brown sugar, 1 ½ cups

- Crystallized ginger, 3 tablespoons

- Bosc pears, 2 firm-ripe

- All-purpose flour, 2 ½ cups

- Baking powder, 2 teaspoons

- Baking soda, 1 teaspoon

- Ground ginger, 1 ½ teaspoons

- Ground cinnamon, 1 teaspoon

- Salt, ½ teaspoon

- Ground allspice, ¼ teaspoon

- Eggs, 2 large

- Dark molasses, ¾ cup

- Buttermilk, 1 ¼ cups

Instructions

1. Start by lightly buttering a 9-inch cake pan with a removable rim measuring 2 1/2 inches in height. Now line the pan with a 10-inch round of cooking parchment paper, pressing the bottom and then 1/2 inches upsides.

2. Then cut 2 tablespoons of butter into the 1/4-inch chunks, drop them evenly over the parchment in the pan bottom.

3. Sprinkle them evenly with a 1/2 cup of brown sugar and also with crystallized ginger.

4. Now peel pears and then cut in half lengthwise, afterward slicing them parallel to cut the edge, cut them into 1/2-inches thick slices. Now with the help of a small knife, tear core from all slices.

5. Now arrange the slices flat, into a single layer, place over the pan's sugar mixture, then trimming the pieces as needed.

6. Whisk in a small bowl, some flour, baking soda, ginger, baking powder, cinnamon, salt, and spices.

7. With the help of an electric mixer, beat together the remaining 1/2 cup of butter and 1 cup of brown sugar until well blended in another bowl. Now add eggs and beat well. Then reduce the speed of the blender to medium-low and then beat in the molasses.

8. Now add the flour mixture and the buttermilk alternately, beat until combined, and then beat again on high speed until well blended. Now pour the batter over the pears.

9. Now bake in 325° convection oven till the toothpick inserted in the center of the cake comes out clean, for 1 hour 35 minutes. Let it cool in the pan on the rack for about 20 min.

10. Now remove the pan sides. Now invert the platter over the cake, hold the two together, then

invert again. Now carefully remove the pan bottom and also the parchment.

11. Serve.

20. Kidney friendly Oat Berry Bars

Calories: 334 kcal| Preparation time: 40 min| Servings: 40 bars |Difficulty: High

Ingredients

Cookie dough:

- Unsalted butter, 1 cup

- Granulated sugar, 1 cup

- Brown sugar packed, 1 cup

- 2 eggs

- Pure vanilla extract, one teaspoon

- All-purpose flour, 1 cup

- Whole wheat flour, 1 cup

- Baking soda, 1 1/2 teaspoon

- Kosher salt, 1 teaspoon

- Ground cinnamon, 1 teaspoon

- Old-fashioned oats, 3 1/2 cups

- Raw quinoa, 1/4 cup

- Shredded unsweetened coconut, 1/2 cup

- Berry mix-in:

- Frozen blackberries, 2 1/2 cups

- Honey, 3 tablespoons

- Half of lemon zest

- Kosher salt, 1/4 teaspoon

- Ground black pepper

Berry glaze:

- Confectioner's sugar, 4 cups

- Pasteurized, 3 egg whites

- Half of lemon zest

- Lemon juice, two tablespoons

- Berry mix-in reserved

Instructions

Cookie dough:

1. In a bowl with a stand mixer having a paddle attachment, mix the butter and some sugar. Now add cream and mix at a medium speed for almost 1 minute.

2. Now add egg, vanilla and cream and mix for 2 minutes on a medium-high.

3. Now add dry ingredients and then mix on low speed until it just gets incorporated. However, do not overmix.

4. Now evenly spread almost 3/4 of the mixture in the half-sized sheet pan. Then distribute prepared berry mix in the cookie mix, now distribute remaining dough all over the fruit.

5. Then bake at the temperature of 325 degrees F in the convection oven for almost 20-25 min till the center is prepared. Cool bars completely, now leave them in the pan. Or you can cool them in the freezer.

6. When you cook them, then pour in the glaze over all the bars, spread with the offset spatula. Now allow frosting to set while keeping it uncovered.

7. Now cut into two by 2-inch squares and then serve.

Berry mix-in preparation:

1. Combine berries, pepper, honey, lemon in a small pot.

2. Then, cook in medium-low heat, stirring it occasionally, and smash the berries with a spoon's back.

3. Now cook for almost 15 minutes or till the mixture gets thicken and berries have broken.

4. Now set them aside to cool, and reserve two tablespoons.

5. Berry glaze preparation:

6. Combine egg whites, lemon juice, lemon zest, also remaining berry mix in the bowl containing a stand mixer with the whisk attachment.

7. Whisk for 30 seconds on medium speed.

8. Add the powdered sugar and beat on low until the sugar is just incorporated.

9. Now on medium speed beat for almost 2 minutes.

10. Glaze finished bars and serve.

21. Peach Pie Rock Creek Lake

Calories: 549 kcal |Preparation time: 40 min | Servings: 8 |Difficulty: Medium

Ingredients

- Pastry

- Cream cheese, 1 package

- Sugar, 1 1/4 cups

- Firm-ripped peaches, 6 1/2 cups

- Orange juice, 3/4 cup

- Cornstarch, 1/4 cup

- Lemon juice, 1/4 cup

Instructions

1. With the help of a fork, prick the bottom and sides of the unbaked pastry in a pan 1-inch apart. Now bake in 375° convection oven till becomes golden, for about 15 to 20 minutes; now let cool on the rack.

2. Now, mix the cream cheese and 1/2 cup of sugar in a bowl until it gets smooth. Then spread it evenly over the bottom of the cool pastry.

3. In a food processor, now whirl in 1 cup of sliced peaches, the remaining 3/4 cup of sugar, some orange juice, and cornstarch until it gets smooth. Now pour into a three by 4-quart pan, stir over in medium-high heat till the mixture boils and thickens for about 4 minutes.

Now remove from the heat and then stir in some lemon juice.

4. Now add the remaining 5 1/2 cups of peaches into the hot peach glaze and then mix and coat the slices. Now let them cool till it is tepid, for about 25 minutes, now scrape them onto the cream cheese mixture's crust.

5. Lastly, chill it uncovered, till it is firm enough to be cut, for 3 hours.

6. Cut into wedge-shaped and then serve

7. It can be inverted in a large bowl over the pie and be chilled up to almost 1 day.

22. Cranberry chocolate chip granola bars

Calories: 181 kcal| Total time: 35mins| Serving 16 | Difficulty: easy)

Ingredients

- Flaked coconut, 1 cup

- Sliced almonds, 1 cup

- Cup pecan halves, 1/2

- Sunflower seeds, 1/2 cup

- Dried cranberries chopped unsweetened, 1/3 cup

- Dark chocolate-chips & sugar-free, 1/3 cup

- Salt ½, teaspoon

- Butter ½, cup

- Yacon syrup, 2 teaspoons

- Swerve sweetener powdered, 1/2 cup

- Vanilla extract, 1/2 teaspoon

23. Sugar-Free Cranberry Sauce

Calories: Kcal 21| Total Time: 20 mins |Serving 8| Difficulty: Easy)

Ingredients

- Bag of cranberries, 12 oz

- Water, 4 oz

- Trim healthy mama sweet, 1 cup

- Vanilla ,1 teaspoon

- Cinnamon, 1 teaspoon

Instructions

1. Stir the cranberries as well as the water in a big saucepan. Cook for around 5 to 7 mins over med heat, until all the berries appear. Bring the rest of the ingredients together & lower the heat to med. Cook until needed fire. Might thicken further as it cools.

2. Put it in the freezer for about 2 weeks.

24. Renal friendly Cranberry Crumb Bars

Calories: Kcal 21| Total Time: 4 hr. |Serving 24| Difficulty: Easy)

Ingredients

- Crust and Topping

- Gold Medal™ 2 1/2

- Cups all-purpose flour

- Sugar, 1 cup

- Ground ½ cup, slivered almonds

- Baking powder, 1 teaspoon

- Salt, ¼ teaspoon

- Cold butter, 1 cup

- 1 egg

- Ground cinnamon, ¼ teaspoon

  Filling

- Fresh or frozen. 4 cups cranberries

- Sugar, 1 cup

- Orange (4 teaspoons) Juice of 1/2

- Cornstarch, 1 Tablespoon

- Vanilla, 1 Teaspoon

Instructions

1. Heat the oven to about 375°F. Now grease pan with some cooking spray.

2. In a big bowl, add flour, sugar, almonds, baking powder and salt. Cut butter until the it looks like crumbs. Add egg and stir. Press this crumb mixture pan's bottom. Stir cinnamon into remaining crumb mixture; set aside.

3. In a separate bowl, stir all ingredients. Spoon it evenly on the crust.

4. Bake for 45 to 55 minutes or until it is light golden brown. Cool and Refrigerate until it is chilled

5. Serve.

25. Apple-cranberry crisps

Calories: 264 kcal| Total Time: 45 minutes | Serves 6 |Difficulty medium

Ingredients

- Apples, 3 medium, cored and chopped

- Cranberries, 1 ½ cups

- Fresh lemon juice 3 tablespoons

- Sugar, 1 tablespoon

- Cinnamon, 1 heaping teaspoon

- Topping

- Oats, 1 ¾ cup

- Flaxseed meal, ¼ cup

- Finely chopped walnuts, 1 cup pecans, optional

- Pure maple syrup, ½ cup

- Coconut oil, 3 – 4 tablespoons

- Vanilla extract, 1 teaspoon

- Mineral salt, ¼ teaspoon

Instructions

1. Preheat the oven to about 350 degrees F.

2. Put all the fruit together with lemon juice, some sugar and cinnamon. Now mix well, then layer into baking dish.

3. In a mixing bowl, combine flaxseed meal, oats, walnuts/pecans, optional coconut oil, maple syrup, vanilla, and salt, then mix well. Spread evenly over apple and cranberries and then sprinkle with more cinnamon.

4. Bake for 35 – 40 minutes, keep an eye on the topping; once done, cool 5 – 10 minutes formerly serving.

5. Serve warm.

Chapter 5: Kidney Friendly Renal Diet Beverages

1. Pineapple-Mint Flavored Water

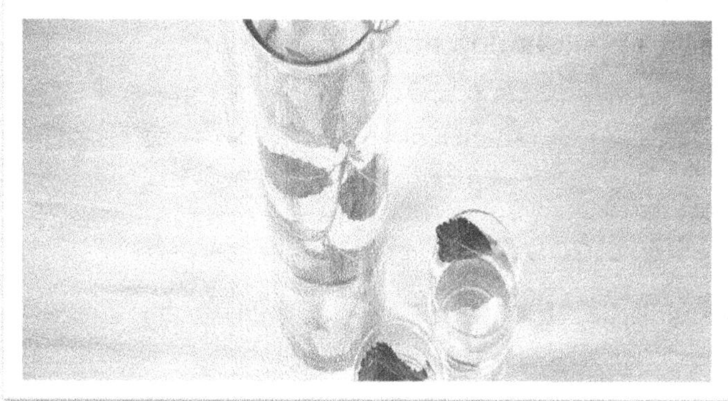

Calories: 10 kcal |Total time: 12 hr. | Serving 8 | Difficulty: Easy

Ingredients

- Fresh pineapple, 1 cup

- Leaves, 12 fresh mint

- Water, 10 cups

Instructions

1. Add all ingredients to a pitcher.

2. Refrigerator overnight

3. Serve.

2. Kidney friendly Mixed Berry Smoothie

Calories: 176 kcal |Total time: 5 min | Serving 2 | Difficulty: Easy

Ingredients

- Very cold water, 4 ounces

- Fresh mixed berries, 1 cup

- Ice cubes, 2

- Crystal liquid flavor, 1 teaspoon

- Whipped cream topping, 1/2 cup

- Whey protein powder. 2 scoops

Instructions

1. Add all ingredients to a blender and mix till combined

2. Serve.

3. Raspberry Milkshake Smoothie

Per serving: 150 Kcal |Total Time: 5 min | Serving: 2 | Difficulty: Easy

Ingredients

- Crushed ice, 1 cup

- Plain almond milk, 1 cup

- Confectioners swerve 2 tablespoon or sweetener of choice

- Cream cheese, 1 tablespoon

- Whipping cream, 1/4 cup

- Raspberries, 1/4 cup

- Vanilla extract, 1/2 teaspoon

- Pinch of table salt (<1/8 teaspoon)

Instructions

1. Mix all of the mentioned ingredients and blend till well-combined.

2. Serve in a glass.

4. Green juice

Calories: 130 kcal| Total Time: 5 minutes | Serving:2 | Difficulty: Easy

Ingredients

- 2 medium, Green apples

- Lemon, 1/2

* 1/2 cup, fresh pineapple

* Cucumber, 1 medium

Instructions

1. Mix all ingredients in a blender till well combined.

2. Serve and enjoy!

5. Kidney friendly Rice milk

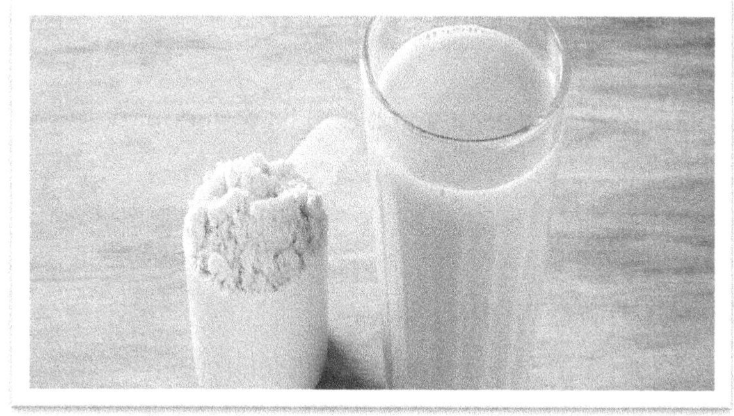

Calories: 130 kcal| Total Time: 5 minutes | Serving: 2| Difficulty: Easy

Ingredients

* Chilled 1 cup, unenriched rice milk

* Vanilla whey protein, 2 scoops

Instructions

1. Blend all ingredients till well combined.

2. Serve in a glass and enjoy it.

6. Vanilla Blackberry Frosted Lemonade

Calories: 183 kcal |Total time: 5 min | Serving 1 | Difficulty: Easy

Ingredients

* Better stevia extract, ½ teaspoon

* Almond unsweetened or cashew milk, 2/3 cup

- Lemon juice, 1/4 cup

- Collagen. 1 tablespoon

- Himalayan or mineral salt, 1 pinch

- Vanilla extract, 1 teaspoon

- Glucomannan, ½ teaspoon

- Blackberries, fresh or frozen 1/2 cup

- Ice cubes, 3 cups

Instructions

1. Mix all of the mentioned ingredients and blend till well-combined.

2. Serve in a glass.

7. Blueberry Coconut Chia Smoothies

Calories: 249 Kcal |Total Time: 5 min | Serving 1 | Difficulty: Easy

Ingredients

- Greek yogurt full fat, 1 cup

- Frozen blueberries, 1 cup

- Coconut cream, 1/2 cup

- Ground chia seed, 2 tablespoons

- swerve sweetener, 2 tablespoons

- Unsweetened almond milk or cashew 1 cup

- Coconut oil, 2 tablespoons

Instructions

1. Mix all of the mentioned ingredients and blend till well-combined.

2. Serve.

8. Coconut Milk Strawberry Smoothie

Calories: 397 Kcal |Total Time: 2 min | Serving 2 | Difficulty: Easy

Ingredients

- Smooth almond butter, 2 tablespoons

- Stevia packets, 2 optional

- Frozen Strawberries, 1 cup

- Unsweetened coconut milk, 1 cup

Instructions

1. Mix all of the mentioned ingredients and blend till well-combined.

2. Serve.

9. Renal friendly Strawberry Milkshake

Calories: 368 kcal| Total Time: 5 min | Serving 1 | Difficulty: Easy

Ingredients

- Coconut Milk, 3/4 cup

- Heavy Cream, 1/4 cup

- Ice Cubes, 7

- Sugar-free Strawberry Torani, 2 tablespoons.

- MCT Oil, 1 tablespoon.

- Xanthan Gum, 1/4 teaspoon.

Instructions

- Mix all of the mentioned ingredients and blend till well-combined.

- Serve in a glass.

10. Simple Blueberry smoothie

Calories: 215 Kcal |Total Time: 5 min | serving 1 | Difficulty: Easy

Ingredients

- Coconut Milk or almond milk, 1 cup

- Blueberries, 1/4 cup

- Vanilla Extract, 1 teaspoon

- MCT Oil or coconut oil, 1 teaspoon

- Protein Powder 30 g optional

Instructions

1. Mix all of the mentioned ingredients and blend till well-combined.

2. Serve in a glass.

11. Blueberry yogurt coconut drink

Calories: 70 Kcal| Total time: 5 min | serving 2 | Difficulty: Easy

Ingredients

- Coconut yogurt ,1 pot (120 ml) of

- Blueberries 10

- Coconut milk ,1 cup

- Vanilla extract, 1/2 teaspoon

- Stevia (taste)

Instructions

1. Mix all of the mentioned ingredients and blend till well-combined.

2. Serve in a glass.

12. Peach Berry Smoothie

Calories: 80 kcal| Total Time: 10 minutes| Serving: 1|Difficulty: Easy

Ingredients:

1. Sea Moss, 1 tablespoon.

2. Coconut Milk, 1 cup

3. Strawberries, ½ cup

4. Hemp Seeds, 1 tablespoon.

5. quartered, Peaches, ½ cup

6. Agave Syrup, 1 tablespoon.

7. Blueberries, ½ cup

Instructions:

1. Mix all of the mentioned ingredients and blend till well-combined.

2. Transfer to the serving glass, drink instantly.

3. Enjoy it!

13. Watermelon Smoothie

Calories: 50 Kcal |Total Time: 10 minutes| Serving: 1|Difficulty: Easy

Ingredients

1. Coconut Water, 1 cup

2. Pieces of Watermelon, 1 cup

3. Date Syrup ,1 tablespoon.

4. Strawberries, 1 cup

Instructions:

1. Start by blending the watermelon and strawberries, then add coconut water and, finally, the dates.

2. Blend till well combined.

3. Transfer to a glass.

4. Enjoy!

14. Apple Smoothie

Calories: 35 kcal| Total Time: 25 min | Serving: 2 |Difficulty: easy

Ingredients:

- Sea Moss, 1 tablespoon.

- Ice, 2 cups

- fresh Apple Juice, 2 cups

- Ginger, 1 tablespoon.

- Clove Powder A Dash

Instructions:

1. Mix all of the mentioned ingredients and blend till well-combined.

2. Now, stir with the ice and blend for another minute.

3. Transfer to the serving glass, drink instantly.

4. Enjoy it!

15. Strawberry Banana Smoothie

Calories: 85 kcal| Total Time: 10 minutes | Serving: 2| Difficulty: Easy

Ingredients:

1. Hemp Milk, 2 cups

2. 4 Banana

3. Dates, ¾ cup

4. Agave, 1 tablespoon.

5. Strawberry, 8 oz.

Instructions:

1. Mix the strawberries and other ingredients in a blender till they are slightly broken down.

2. Then add banana and hemp milk. Put agave. Blend till well mixed.

3. Serve and enjoy it!

16. Apple-Cinnamon Flavored Water

Calories: 4 kcal| Total Time: 12 hrs. | Serving: 8 | Difficulty: Easy

Ingredients

1. Water, 10 cups

2. Apple, 1 medium

3. Sticks, 2 cinnamon

4. Ground cinnamon, 2 teaspoons

Instructions

1. Cut a peeled apple into slices and soak all ingredients in water

2. Refrigerate overnight.

3. Serve

17. Beet and Apple Juice Blend

Calories: 53 kcal| Total Time: 5 minutes | Serving: 2 | Difficulty: Easy

Ingredients

- Apple, 1/2 medium

- Beet, 1/2 medium

- fresh carrot, 1 medium

- stalk, 1 celery

- parsley, 1/4 cup

Instructions

1. Put all ingredients in a juicer and extract the juice.

2. Transfer to a glass.

3. Enjoy!

18. Blackberry-Sage Flavored Water

Calories: 7 kcal| Total Time: 12 hrs. | Serving: 8 | Difficulty: Easy

Ingredients

- Fresh blackberries, 1 cup
- Sage leaves, 4
- Water, 10 cups

Instructions

1. Mash blackberries and add all ingredients to a pitcher.
2. Refrigerator overnight.
3. Serve and enjoy.

19. Blueberry Blast Smoothie

Calories: 108 kcal| Total Time: minutes | Serving: | Difficulty: Easy

Ingredients

- Frozen blueberries, 1 cup
- Splenda® ,8 packets
- Protein powder, 6 tablespoons
- Ice cubes ,8
- Apple juice, 14 ounces

Instructions

1. Mix all of the mentioned ingredients and blend till well-combined.
2. Serve in a glass.

20. Café au Lait Protein Wake-Up

Calories: 100 kcal| Total Time: 5 minutes | Serving: 1| Difficulty: Easy

Ingredients

1. Protein powder, 1 scoop

2. Hot coffee ,8 ounces

3. Flavored liquid ,2 tablespoons coffee creamer

Instructions

1. Place one scoop of protein powder in a cup. Add coffee and stir until dissolved.

2. Now add coffee creamer.

3. Serve and enjoy.

21. Caramel Protein Latte

Calories: 72 kcal| Total Time: 5 minutes | Serving: 1 | Difficulty: Easy

Ingredients

- Whey protein powder, 1 scoop

- Water, 2 ounces

- Hot coffee, 6 ounces

- Caramel syrup Sugar-Free, 2 tablespoons

Instructions

1. Transfer protein powder in a jug, add water and mix till dissolved.

2. Now add hot coffee and stir.

3. Now add caramel syrup.

4. Serve in a cup and enjoy.

22. Kidney friendly Chocolate Smoothie

Calories: 215 kcal| Total Time: minutes | Serving: | Difficulty: Easy

Ingredients

- Powered Bakers Cocoa, 1 tablespoon unsweetened

- Cold water, 1 tablespoon

- Sugar, 1 tablespoon

- Egg white, 8 ounces

- Whipped topping, 4 tablespoons

- Chocolate bar shavings

Instructions

1. Mix cocoa, sugar, and water. Add and mix egg whites and whipping cream till combined.

2. Serve

23. High Protein Berry Shake

Calories: 179 kcal| Total Time: 5 minutes | Serving: 3 | Difficulty: Easy

Ingredients

- Sherbet, 1/2 cup

- Low-cholesterol, 1/4 cup egg product

- Soy milk, 1/2 cup

- Whey protein powder, 3 tablespoons

- Cranberry juice, 1/4 cup

- Frozen blueberries, 1/2 cup

- 2 ice cubes

Instructions

1. Blend all ingredients till well combined.

2. Serve in a glass and enjoy it.

24. Fabulous Hot Cocoa

Calories:72 kcal| Total Time: 10 minutes | Serving: 1 | Difficulty: Easy

Ingredients

- Hot water, 1 cup

- Cocoa powder, 1tablespoon

- Sugar, 2 tablespoons

- Coldwater, 2 tablespoons

- Whipped cream, 2 tablespoons

Instructions

1. Mix cocoa powder & sugar and add cold water to make a thin paste.

2. Now add hot water and stir.

3. Top with some whipped cream.

4. Serve.

25. Peach Pineapple Fruit Smoothie

Calories: 200 kcal| Total Time: 5 minutes | Serving: 1 | Difficulty: Easy

Ingredients

- Canned pineapple, 1/2 cup

- Peaches, 1/2 cup

- Just whites®, 2 tablespoons

- Sugar, 1 tablespoon

Instructions

1. Mix all of the mentioned ingredients and blend till well-combined.

2. Serve in a glass.

26. Strawberry-Apple Juice Blend

Calories: 84 kcal| Total Time: 5 minutes | Serving: 2 | Difficulty: Easy

Ingredients

- Strawberries, 1 cup

- Apple, 1 medium

- Mint leaves ,6

- Lemon, 1/4

- Green tea, 4 ounces

Instructions

1. Mix all berries, lemon and mint and extract juice, add tea.

2. Serve in a glass.

27. Kidney friendly Spooky punch

Calories: 28 kcal| Total Time: 2 hrs. | Serving: 20 | Difficulty: Easy

Ingredients

- Diet 7UP®, 2 liters

- Orange liquid, 5 teaspoons

- Orange sherbet, 1 pint

Instructions

1. Mix all ingredients and refrigerate for an hour.

2. Serve.

28. Spicy eggnog

Calories:162 kcal| Total Time: 5 minutes | Serving: 2 | Difficulty: Easy

Ingredients

- Half & half creamer, 2 cups

- Low cholesterol, 3/4 cup egg product

- Sugar, 1/4 cup

- Rum extract, 2 teaspoons

- Pumpkin pie spice, 1/2 teaspoon

- Nutmeg, 1/4 teaspoon

- Whipped cream, 6 tablespoons

Instructions

1. Mix all of the mentioned ingredients and blend till well-combined.

2. Serve in a glass.

29. Snow cone smoothies

Calories:118 kcal| Total Time: 5 minutes | Serving: 1 | Difficulty: Easy

Ingredients

- Kool-Aid® liquid ,1 teaspoon strawberry flavor drops

- pasteurized liquid, 8 ounces egg white

- Reddi-Wip® dairy, 3 tablespoons whipped topping

Instructions

1. Mix all of the mentioned ingredients and blend till well-combined.

2. Serve in a glass.

30. Strawberry Dreamsicle Delight

Calories:129 kcal| Total Time: 5 minutes | Serving: 4 | Difficulty: Easy

Ingredients

- Almond milk, 2 cups

- Whey protein powder, 3 scoops

- Vanilla syrup, 1/4 cup

- Strawberry extract, 2 teaspoons

- Strawberry soda, 1/2 cup

Instructions

1. Mix all of the mentioned ingredients and blend till well-combined.

2. Serve in a glass.

Chapter 6: Kidney Friendly Renal Diet Salads

1. Cucumber and Radish Salad

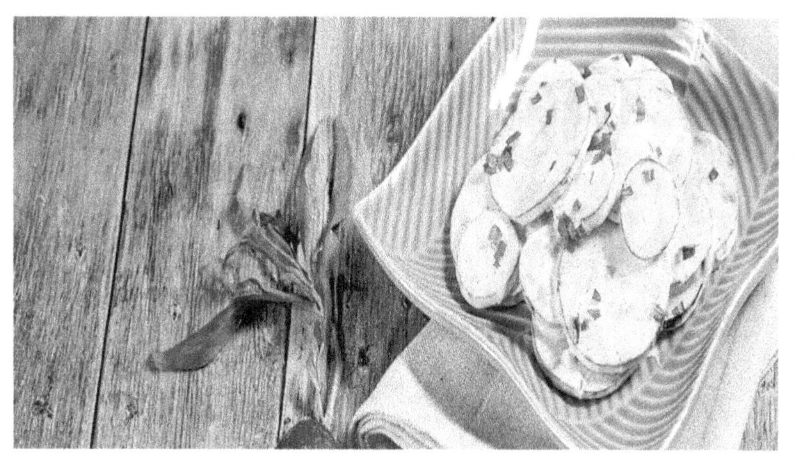

Calories: 60 kcal| Total time: 25 minutes| Servings: 4|Difficulty: Easy

Ingredients

- Garlic, 1 clove, minced

- Fresh tarragon, 2 sprigs, chopped

- Cucumber, 1 large, sliced

- Red radishes, 12 large, sliced

- White wine vinegar, 1 teaspoon

- Light sour cream, 1/2 cup

- Ground black pepper, 1/2 teaspoon

Instructions

1. In a bowl, mix all ingredients.

2. Refrigerator for 20 minutes.

3. Serve

2. Kidney friendly Cranberry salad

Calories: 78 kcal| Total time: 15 minutes| Servings: 8|Difficulty: Easy

Ingredients

- Raw cranberries, 1-1/3 cups

- Sugar, 1/3 cup

- Miniature marshmallows, 1-1/3 cups

- Canned pineapple, 2/3 cup chunks in juice

- Whipped topping, 2/3 cup

Instructions

1. Grind cranberries and sugar in the grinder. Let stand and drain.

2. Dice pineapple chunks.

3. Add both marshmallows and pineapple in cranberries.

4. Serve in a glass.

---

3. Dijon Salad Dressing

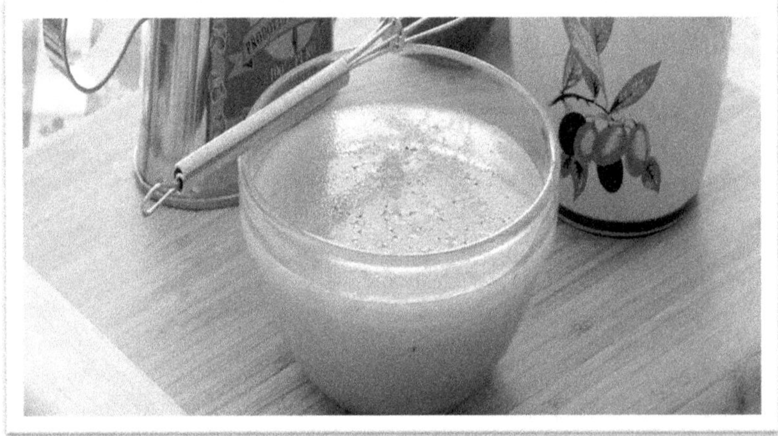

Calories: 78 kcal| Total time: 15 minutes Servings: 8|Difficulty: Easy

Ingredients

- Dijon mustard, 2 tablespoons

- Olive oil, 1/4 cup

- Unseasoned rice vinegar, 1/3 cup

- Brown sugar, 1 tablespoon

* Herb seasoning blend, 1 teaspoon

Instructions

1. Combine all ingredients and stir until it is mixed.

2. Chill and Serve.

4. Kidney friendly Fruit salad slaw

Calories: 115 kcal| Total time: 15 minutes| Servings: 6|Difficulty: Easy

Ingredients

* Red apples, diced

* Purple cabbage, 1/2 cup, shredded

* Green cabbage, 1/2 cup, cut

* Carrots, grated, 1/4 cup

* Canned crushed pineapple, 8 ounces

* Mayonnaise, 1/4 cup

* Pineapple juice, 3 tablespoons

* Sugar, 2 teaspoons

Instructions

1. Blend mayonnaise, pineapple juice and sugar. Set aside.

2. In a separate medium bowl, transfer pineapple, cabbage, carrots, and apples.

3. Add mayonnaise mixture and mix.

4. Refrigerate

5. Serve.

5. Kidney friendly Jicama Fabulous

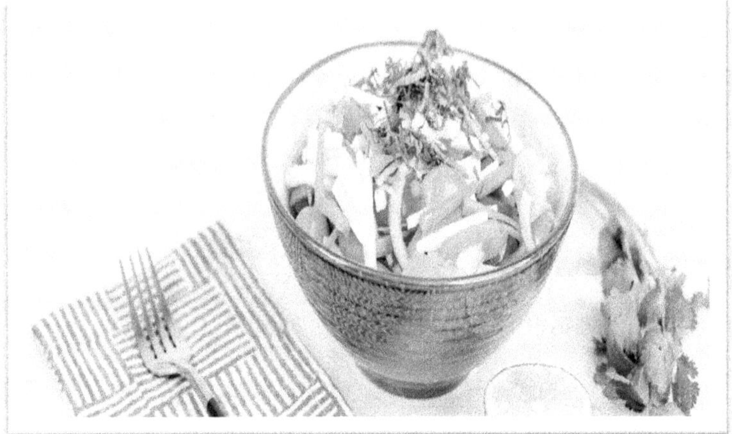

Calories: 52 kcal| Total time: 15 minutes| Servings: 10|Difficulty: Easy

Ingredients

- Jicama, 1 medium peeled, matchstick cuts, 1/4-inch

- Carrot, 1 large peeled, matchstick cuts 1/4-inch

- Red onion, 1/2 medium, diced

- Seedless grapes, 1-1/2 cup, cut in half

- Fresh basil leaves 1/3 cup, small pieces

- Apple cider vinegar, 2 tablespoons

- Lemon juice, 3 tablespoons

- Lime juice, 3 tablespoons

Instructions

1. Add all ingredients to a bowl.

2. Mix and chill.

3. Serve and enjoy.

6. Summer Salad

Calories: 24 kcal| Total time: 15 minutes Servings: 4|Difficulty: Easy

Ingredients

- Tomato, chopped, 1 medium

- Cucumber, sliced, 1/4 medium

- Iceberg lettuce, shred, 3 cups

- Carrot, shred, 1 medium

Instructions

1. Transfer vegetables to bowl and mix.

2. Chill.

3. Serve.

7. Kidney friendly Tabbouleh Salad

Calories: 182 kcal| Total time: 15 minutes| Servings: 8|Difficulty: Easy

Ingredients

- Dry bulgur, 1/2 cup

- Tomato, 1 medium, diced

- Cucumber, 1 medium, chopped

- Green onions, 1 bunch, chopped

- Parsley, 2 bunches, chopped

- Mint, 1/2 bunch, chopped

- Olive oil, 1/2 cup

- lemons, 3 juice

- Salt, 1/2 teaspoon

- Black pepper, 1/2 teaspoon

Instructions

1. Wash bulgur and drain. Then pour boiling water over the bulgur and cover it.

2. Let it sit for about 30 minutes and drain.

3. Add vegetables and add remaining ingredients to the bulgur mixture.

4. Let it sit for about an hour.

5. Serve.

8. Iceberg Wedge Salad

Calories: 201 kcal| Total time: 15 minutes| Servings: 4|Difficulty: Easy

Ingredients

for dressing-

- Worcestershire dash

- Blue cheese, crumbles, ¼ c

- Plain Greek yogurt, ¼ c

- Sour cream, 3 tablespoons

- Mayonnaise 1 tablespoon

- Milk 3 tablespoon

- White balsamic vinegar, 2 teaspoons

- Salt & pepper >>to taste

For the wedge's salads-

- One iceberg lettuce cut into 4

- Bacon cooked & crumbled, 1/3 cup

- Grape tomatoes, sliced in half, 10

- Extra blue cheese crumbled, 1-2 tablespoon per salad

- Chives

- Hard-boiled eggs, chopped, 4

Instructions

1. Whisk all ingredients together in a small bowl. Put aside.

2. Place wedges of iceberg lettuce on two diner plates cut side up.

3. Gently drizzle with dressing.

4. Top with bacon, eggs, tomatoes, chives, and extra blue cheese.

5. Serve

9. Kidney friendly Cauliflower Salad

Calories: 102 kcal| Total time: 15 minutes| Servings: 8|Difficulty: Easy

Ingredients

- Raw cauliflower, 2 cups, chopped

- Radicchio, ½ cup, chopped

- Artichoke hearts, ½ cup, chopped

- Fresh basil, 1/3 cup, chopped

- Parmesan, ½ cup, grated

- Sundried tomatoes, 3 tablespoons, chopped

- Kalamata olives, 3 tablespoons, chopped

- Clove Garlic, 1, minced

- Balsamic vinegar, 3 tablespoons

- Olive oil, 3 tablespoons

- Salt & pepper

Instructions

1. First, bake the chopped cauliflower for five minutes in the microwave. Cool down the cauliflower.

2. In a medium bowl, combine the artichoke heart, radicchio, basil, parmesan, olives, sundried tomatoes, & garlic.

3. Whisk the vinegar and olive oil together in a small bowl and then pour over salad.

4. Toss it to coat, and sprinkle with salt & pepper.

5. Serve

10. Strawberry jello salad

Calories: 255 kcal| Total time: 10 minutes| Servings: 10|Difficulty: Easy

Ingredients

- 4% fat large curd cottage cheese, 1 cup

- Heavy whipping cream, 1 cup

- Vanilla extract, unsweetened, ½ teaspoon

- Mascarpone cheese softened, 8 oz

- Chopped walnuts, ¼ cup

- Sugar-free strawberry jello, 6 oz

- Unsweetened shredded coconut, 1/3 cup

- Chopped strawberries, 2 cups

Instructions

1. Beat the heavy whipping cream & vanilla in a medium bowl. Fold in the mascarpone cheese carefully until fully incorporated. Gently stir in jello-free cottage cheese & powdered sugar, then mix well.

2. Fold in walnuts, coconut & strawberries.

3. Dip the container in hot water for about twenty seconds to unmold, and then flip over to a serving platter.

4. Store leftovers in the refrigerator in an airtight container for up to 5 days

5. Serve

11. Peanut Sauce topped Noodles salad

Calories: 212 kcal| Total time: 10 minutes| Servings: 4|Difficulty: Easy

Ingredients

For the salad:

- Shredded red cabbage, 1 cup

- Shredded green cabbage, 1 cup

- Shirataki noodles, 4 cups

- Chopped peanuts, ¼ cup

- Chopped scallions, ¼ cup

- Chopped cilantro, ¼ cup

For the dressing:

- Minced ginger, 2 tablespoons

- Cayenne pepper, ¼ teaspoon

- Kosher salt, ½ teaspoon

- Granulated erythritol sweetener, 1 tablespoon

- Toasted sesame oil, 1 tablespoon

- Minced garlic, 1 teaspoon

- Filtered water, ½ cup

- Lime juice, 1 tablespoon

- Wheat-free soy sauce, 1 tablespoon

- Fish sauce, 1 tablespoon

- Sugar-free peanut butter, ¼ cup

Instructions

1. Combine all the ingredients for the salad in a large bowl.

2. Combine all the ingredients for the dressing in a blender. Mix till smooth.

3. Pour the salad over the dressing & toss to coat.

4. Serve immediately.

5. Enjoy.

12. Broccoli plus apple salad

Calories: 287 kcal| Total time: 10 minutes| Servings: 8|Difficulty: Easy

Ingredients

- Broccoli, 6 cups

- Red vinegar, 2 tablespoons

- Chopped cooked bacon, 8 slices

- Chopped onion, 1/3 cup

- Mayonnaise, 1 cup

- Chopped Almonds, ½ cup

- Salt & pepper

Instructions

1. Combine broccoli, bacon, onion & almonds in a large bowl.

2. Mix mayonnaise, vinegar, salt & pepper in a separate bowl, then in a small bowl.

3. Pour broccoli mixture over the dressing and stir.

4. Cover and chill.

5. Serve.

13. Kidney friendly Eggplant towers

Calories: 558 kcal| Total time: 40 minutes| Servings: 4|Difficulty: Easy

Ingredients

- Eggplant, 1

- Fresh mozzarella cheese, 9 oz

- Tomatoes, 2

- Olive oil, 2 tablespoons

- Fresh basil, 8 oz

- Olive oil, ½ cup

- Balsamic vinegar, 1.5 tablespoon

- Garlic clove, 1

- Salt, ½ teaspoon

- Ground black pepper >>to taste

- Fresh basil, 5 oz

- Cherry tomatoes, 4 oz

Instructions

Eggplant towers

1. Cut in 1⁄2 "(1 cm) slices of eggplant, mozzarella, and tomato.

2. Heat the olive oil over medium heat in a frying pan & fry the eggplant till golden.

3. Place an eggplant slice in each plate's center to assemble the platter, then add a slice of mozzarella accompanied by a tomato slice.

4. Add the basil dressing in a spoonful.

5. Continue processing on single plates until all ingredients have been used, approximately 6 slices per tower.

6. Complete your creations with a bit more basil dressing over the top and scatter some cherry tomatoes halves around the plate.

Basil dressing

1. Place the basil, garlic, salt, and olive oil in a food processor for basil dressing and blend until smooth.

14. Crispy Kidney friendly cucumber salad

Calories: 27 kcal| Total time: 10 minutes| Servings: 4|Difficulty: Easy

Ingredients

- Fresh cucumber, 2 cups, ¼-inch slices

- Caesar salad dressing, 2 tablespoons

- Ground black pepper as desired

Directions

1. In a bowl, combine cucumber with salad dressing.

2. Cover the bowl with a lid and shake it to coat.

3. Sprinkle it with black pepper.

4. Refrigerate and serve.

15. Lemon Orzo Spring Salad

Calories: 330 kcal| Total time: 40 minutes| Servings: 4|Difficulty: Easy

Ingredients

- Orzo pasta, ¾ cup

- Fresh yellow peppers, ¼ cup, diced

- Fresh red peppers, ¼ cup, diced

- Fresh green peppers, ¼ cup, diced

- Fresh red onion, ½ cup, diced

- Fresh zucchini, 2 cups, medium-cubed

- Olive oil, ¼ cup

- Fresh lemon juice, 3 tablespoons

- Lemon zest, 1 teaspoon

- Grated parmesan cheese, 3 tablespoons

- Fresh rosemary, 2 tablespoons, chopped

- Black pepper, ½ teaspoon

- Dried oregano, ½ teaspoon

- Red pepper flakes, ½ teaspoon

Instructions

- Cook orzo pasta as directed on the box and drain.

- On medium-high heat, sauté peppers, zucchini, and onions with oil in a pan until translucent.

- Now mix lemon juice, cheese, rosemary, lemon zest, olive oil, pepper, oregano, red pepper in a bowl.

- Add vegetables and pasta into the bowl and fold it until well combined.

- Chill and serve.

16. Shrimp and Veggie Noodle Salad

Calories: 254 kcal| Total time: 50 minutes| Servings: 10|Difficulty: Medium

Ingredients

- Dry Spaghetti, 1-pound package, cooked

- Cooked cocktail shrimp, 4 cups

- Fresh scallions, sliced, 1 cup

- Fresh broccoli florets, 2 cups

- Fresh carrots, shredded, 1 cup

- Shitake mushrooms, chopped, 2 cups

- Sesame oil, 2 tablespoons

- Chili oil, 2 teaspoons

- Rice wine vinegar, ½ cup

- Fresh garlic, chopped, 2 tablespoons

- Fresh ginger, chopped, 1 tablespoon

- Soy sauce, low sodium, ¼ cup

- Lime juice, ¼ cup

Instructions

1. Transfer 1 cup soy sauce substitute in a saucepan.

2. Mix the first six ingredients in a bowl; set aside.

3. Blend other ingredients in the blender for about 1 minute.

4. Now pour dressing mixture on pasta mixture. Mix to coat well.

5. Serve

17. Crunchy Quinoa salad

Calories: 158 kcal| Total time: 40 minutes| Servings: 8|Difficulty: Easy

Ingredients

- Quinoa, 1 cup, rinsed
- Water, 2 cups
- Cherry tomatoes, diced, 5
- Cucumbers, ½ cup, seeded and diced
- Onions, chopped, 3 green
- Fresh mint, chopped, ¼ cup
- Parsley, chopped, ½ cup
- Fresh lemon juice, 2 tablespoons
- Grated lemon rind, 1 tablespoon
- Olive oil, 4 tablespoons
- Parmesan cheese, grated, ¼ cup
- Lettuce, ½ head

Instructions

1. Toast quinoa in pan on medium-high heat, stirring frequently. Add water and boil. Reduce heat and cover the pan, and simmer. Cool it.

2. Combine all remaining ingredients in a bowl. Add the cooled quinoa to the mixture.

3. Spoon mixture in the lettuce cups and sprinkle parmesan on top.

4. Serve and enjoy.

18. Mashed Squash Salad

Calories: 90 kcal| Total time: 10 minutes| Servings: 6|Difficulty: Easy

Ingredients:

- Allspice, 1 teaspoon.

- Blue Agave, ¼ cup, natural

- Squash 2, skinned & cubed

- Sea Salt, 1/8 teaspoon.

- Date Sugar, ¼ cup

- Hemp Milk, ¼ cup

Directions

1. Put the squash chunks and the water in a saucepan over medium flame.

2. Boil the mixture and simmer for twenty minutes or when the squash is soft.

3. When soft, drain the water, then mash the squash.

4. After this, add a spoon of date sugar, organic milk, spice, sea salt and agave. Mix it well.

5. Serve yourself and love it.

19. Chickpeas Salad

Calories: 558 kcal| Total time: 40 minutes| Servings: 4|Difficulty: Easy

Ingredients:

- Chickpeas, 1 ½ cups, washed

- Red onion, ½ cup, cubed

- Cilantro, ¼ cup, fresh one & well chopped

- Avocado, 1 cup

- Sea salt as per taste

Directions

1. First, put the chickpeas in a bowl and mash it with the masher.

2. Add the avocado and then mix it properly.

3. In this mixture, add lemon juice and blend properly. Then whisk with the lime juice, blend, and mix with the cilantro. Stir it again. Then, add a spoon of salt. Whisk it again.

4. Serve and enjoy yourself

20. Fetish Mango Salad

Calories: 558 kcal| Total time: 45 minutes| Servings: 4|Difficulty: Easy

Ingredients:

- Mangoes, 2

- Red onion, 1/4

- Cherry tomatoes, 1/4 cup

- Cucumber 1/2, having seeds

- Bell pepper ½, green

- Key lime, 1

- Sea salt according to taste

- Cayenne pepper according to taste

Directions:

Preparing Mango Salad begins with cutting the mangoes, chopping the red onion, and slicing the cherry tomatoes. Slice thinly the seeded cucumber as well as the bell pepper. In a little tub, add all the ingredients and mix. Take the lime and spill over the salad.

Sprinkle with salt and cayenne pepper and leave for marinating in the refrigerator for about 20 minutes before feeding. Enjoy it as your salad, salsa or even a dip; that is your call!

21. Kidney friendly Strawberry and dandelion Salad

Calories: 250 kcal| Total time: 50 minutes| Servings: 4|Difficulty: Easy

Ingredients:

- Grape-seed oil, 2 tablespoons

- Strawberries, 10, chopped

- Red onion, 1 medium, chopped

- Dandelion greens, 4 cups

- Key lime juice, 2 tablespoons

- Sea salt as per taste

Directions:

1. Take a nonstick pan, put grape-seed oil in it, heat it over medium flame. Add sea salt and the sliced onions to the pan. Cook and stir regularly until the onions are smooth, softly golden.

2. In a cup, add lime juice to the strawberry slices.

3. Clean the dandelion greens and break them into bite-sized bits.

4. Once the onions are almost done, pour the rest of the key lime juice into the pan, then cook for a few minutes till the onions are browned.

5. Remove from heat. In the salad bowl, mix the onions, greens, and strawberries along with all of the juices. Sprinkle the sea salt.

6. Serve and enjoy.

22. Grilled Vegetable Pasta Salad

Calories: 377 kcal| Total time: 50 minutes| Servings: 8|Difficulty: Easy

Ingredients

- Garlic cloves, minced, 2

- Gijon mustard, 1 tablespoon

- Lemon juice, 1/4 cup)

- Olive oil, 1/4 cup

- Black pepper, 1/2 teaspoon

- Rotini, uncooked, 12 ounces

- Zucchini, sliced, 2 meds

- Head anise, sliced, 1

- Quartered mushrooms, 8

- Red onion, sliced, 1 med

- Fresh basil leaves, shredded, 2 tablespoons

- Fresh thyme, 1 tablespoon

- Fresh parsley, chopped, 1 tablespoon

Instructions

1. Make the dressing by adding all the ingredients in a mixing bowl together and whisking them together,

2. All vegetables are added to a big mixing bowl. Pour half of the dressing over the vegetables and mix until they are all finely coated. Allow the vegetables to marinate when cooking the pasta according to the package directions. In cool water, rinse the noodles.

3. Turn the oven on to broil in the meantime or start cooking up the barbeque. If the oven is used, use the greased broiler pan, or use the grill basket if using the barbeque.

4. Spread the vegetables on the broiling pan or the hot grill basket the vegetable mixture and cook until the vegetables become golden brown. To allow the browning to occur uniformly, stir them after every 4-5 mins. Pour in a serving bowl when browned, add the pasta & the leftover dressing, and add the fresh herbs. Toss, then serve.

---

23. Kidney friendly citrus salad

Calories: 106 kcal| Total time: 15 minutes| Servings: 8|Difficulty: Easy

Ingredients

- Blood oranges, peeled and pith removed, 20 ounces

- Extra-virgin olive oil, 2 tablespoons

- Kalamata olives pitted & halved, ¼ cup

- Fresh rosemary, roughly chopped, 2 tablespoons

- White wine or champagne vinegar, 1 tablespoon

- Red onion, sliced, 2 tablespoons

- Pomegranate seeds, 2 tablespoons

- Sea salt, ¼ teaspoon

Instructions

1. Cut into rounds the oranges crosswise.

2. On a serving plate, Arrange orange slices.

3. Heat the oil for approximately 1 min in a small skillet over med-high heat. Lower the heat to med.

4. Olives & rosemary are added. Cook and mix till the rosemary sizzle for around 2 minutes, mildly, but green.

5. Take it off the heat and pour it into a little bowl.

6. Stir immediately in the vinegar. Add slices of onion.

7. Pour the mixture of dressing over the oranges.

8. If needed, season it with sea salt.

9. Garnish and serve with pomegranate seeds.

24. Red Cabbage with Apples

Calories: 67 kcal| Total time: 45 minutes| Servings: 6|Difficulty: Easy

Ingredients

- Coarsely chopped, 1 onion

- Olive or vegetable oil, 2 tablespoons

- Cider vinegar, 1/4 cup

- Brown sugar, 2 tablespoons

- Green apple, 1

- Head red cabbage, 1 small

Instructions

1. Sauté the onion in the oil in a broad skillet until softened (nearly 5 minutes).

2. Add the vinegar, sugar & pepper. Add the apple and cabbage.

3. Carry to a boil, lower the heat, cover, and simmer, stirring periodically, until the cabbage wilts (about 10 minutes).

4. Serve.

25. Kidney friendly strawberry wedge salad

Calories: 100 kcal| Total time: 35 minutes| Servings: 4|Difficulty: Easy

Ingredients

- Strawberries washed and halved, 1 cup

- Salt-free garlic powder, 1/4 teaspoon

- Salt-free chipotle powder, 1/4 teaspoon

- Olive oil, 3 tablespoons

- Sour cream, 1/2 cup

- Freshly ground black pepper

- Handful dill, finely chopped

- Head of butter lettuce, leaves washed and separated

Instructions

1. Set it to 375o F in the oven.

2. Mix the strawberries with a tablespoon of oil & the garlic & chipotle powder in a bowl. Using the hands till the strawberries are coated nicely, to mix gently. Then use parchment paper to cover an oven sheet to spread out the strawberry slices in a single layer. Place the mixture in the oven & roast for 12-15 minutes.

3. Add the sour cream, pepper, the remaining two tablespoon of oil, and one tablespoon of water to another bowl for the dressing. Use a fork/whisk to mix once you have developed a milky dressing. Add some splash of water if it is already too dense until it has a perfect consistency. Then add the dill & give it another soft whirl before all the green bits are added.

4. For family-style, put the leaves on plates (individual) or on one wide serving platter. Drizzle over the leaves with your dressing and put on top the chipotle strawberries.

26. Violet Green Salad

Calories: 105 kcal| Total time: 15 minutes| Servings: 4|Difficulty: Easy

Ingredients

- Spring greens, 4 cups

- Cucumber,1

- Sugar snap peas or frozen peas, 1 cup

- Pear, 1

- Goat cheese,3 oz

- Chive flowers, violets or edible flowers, 1 oz

- Plain or Greek plain yogurt, 1/4 cup

- Pomegranate molasses, 1/4 cup

- Lemon Juice, 2 tablespoons

- Fresh parsley, 1/4 cup

- Olive oil, 1/2 cup

- Mustard, 1 teaspoon

- Pinch, 1

- Nuts, optional, 1/4 cup

Instructions

1. Tear greens into pieces that are bite-size.

2. Cut the cucumber into discs and quarters.

3. If you use frozen peas, into thirds split snap peas in pods, let them thaw for about half an hour at room temp.

4. Dice the pear & combine it with the greens.

5. If you've some, combine the goat cheese to chives, then break or part in 1/2-inch bits.

6. Mix the yogurt, lemon juice, molasses, parsley, allspice olive oil, and mustard in a food processor or blender.

7. Toss the salad with the dressing.

8. For a perfect presentation, disperse goat cheese, flowers & nuts over the top.

27. Kidney friendly beet salad

Calories: 308 kcal| Total time: 1 hr. 5 minutes| Servings: 4|Difficulty: Medium

Ingredients

- Chilled beets, roasted, peeled, and diced, 4

- Walnuts or pecans, 1/2 cup

- Leaf lettuce, 1

- Olive oil, 2 tablespoons

- Stilton or blue cheese, 2-3 ounce.

- Fresh basil, chopped fine, 1/4 cup

- Fruit or herb vinegar, 1/2 cup

Instructions

1. Heat the oven to 400°.

2. Roast beets till soft, 45 min. Approx.

3. Chill, dice, and peel.

4. In a saucepan, add the nuts, water, and sugar. The mixture is heated, stirring continually until most of the liquid bubbles are eliminated.

5. Pour nuts on aluminum foil or parchment paper when nuts are coated, & the frying pan is nearly dry. Separate nuts when still hot.

6. Let it cool, and it can be kept for many months at room temperature.

7. Prepare a bed of lettuce.

8. Toss the beets with vinegar, basil, and oil.

9. Sprinkle it on a bed of lettuce.

10. Scatter cheese pieces and nuts all over the top.

28. Blueberry and wild rice salad

Calories: 250 kcal| Total time: 35 minutes| Servings: 8|Difficulty: Easy

Ingredients

- Wild rice, 1 cup
- Water, 2 cups
- Collard greens, lightly steamed, 1 cup
- Onion, chopped, 1/2 cup
- Mixed berries, 2 1/2 cups
- Blueberries, 1/4 cup
- Lemon Juice, 2 tablespoons
- Fresh mint, chopped, 1/4 cup
- Olive oil, 1 tablespoon
- Reduced-fat sour cream, 1/2 cup

Instructions

1. Put the water and rice in a wide saucepan.
2. Bring to a boil, lower heat to low, cover and simmer for 45-55 mins or till most of the liquid has been absorbed.
3. Empty the rice and add the steamed greens, onions, and berries to a wide mixing cup.
4. Mix thoroughly.
5. Purée all the dressing ingredients besides sour cream in a food processor or blender until it is well mixed, incorporating further liquid if needed.
6. Whisk the sour cream gently until well combined.
7. Pour the dressing over the rice salad and coat it with a toss.
8. Serve promptly or place for later usage wrapped it in the refrigerator.

29. Raspberry and Vinegar salad

Calories: 90 kcal| Total time: 5 minutes| Servings: 4|Difficulty: Easy

Ingredients

- Raspberry vinegar, 1/2 cup

- Oil ,1/4 cup

- Dijon mustard ,1 teaspoon

- Sugar ,1 tablespoon

- Mint leaves, chopped, 1/4 cup

Instructions

1. In a tiny bowl, mix all the ingredients together.

2. Serve.

30. Creamy Fruit Salad

Calories: 261 kcal| Total time: 10 minutes| Servings: 8|Difficulty: Easy

Ingredients

- Strawberries, cut in quarters, lengthwise, 1 cup

- Blueberries, 1 cup

- Peaches, diced, 2 meds

- Plain Greek yogurt, 1 cup

- Brown sugar cinnamon, to taste 2 teaspoons

- Lemon, juiced, 1

Instructions

1. In a med mixing bowl, bring all the fruit in.

2. In a little bowl, combine the yogurt, lemon juice, and brown cinnamon sugar. Mix thoroughly.

3. Add the mixture of yogurt to the fruit. Combine, modify the seasoning as required and enjoy

4. Leftovers can be held for about 2 days, refrigerated.

Chapter 7: Kidney Friendly Renal Diet Snacks

1. Simple Pineapple with chili

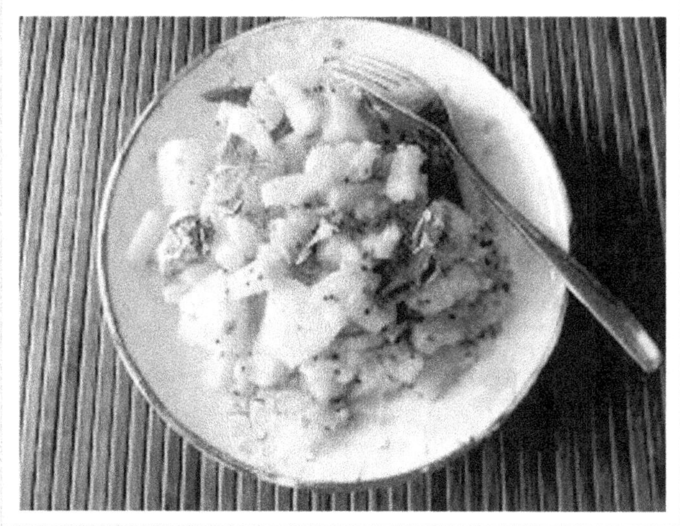

Calories: 88 kcal| Total time: 2 minutes| Servings: 1|Difficulty: Easy

Ingredients

- Pineapple chunks, fresh, 1 cup
- Chili flakes, ½ tablespoon

Instructions

1. Transfer pineapple to a medium-sized bowl.
2. Sprinkle pineapple with chili flakes and enjoy.

2. Kidney friendly Herbed Biscuits

Calories: 109 kcal| Total time: 20 minutes| Servings: 12|Difficulty: Easy

Ingredients

- All-purpose flour, 1¾ cups
- Cream of tartar, 1 teaspoon
- Baking soda, ½ teaspoon
- Mayonnaise, ¼ cup

- Skim milk, ⅔ cup

- Chives, 3 tablespoons, fresh

Instructions

1. Preheat the oven to 400° F.

2. Spray cookie sheet with cooking spray.

3. In a bowl, add flour, cream, baking soda and mayonnaise and mix until the mixture looks like cornmeal.

4. In a separate bowl, add milk, herbs, and flour mixture. Stir.

5. Place on the cookie sheet and bake for almost 10 minutes.

6. Refrigerate.

7. Serve.

3. Roasted grapes

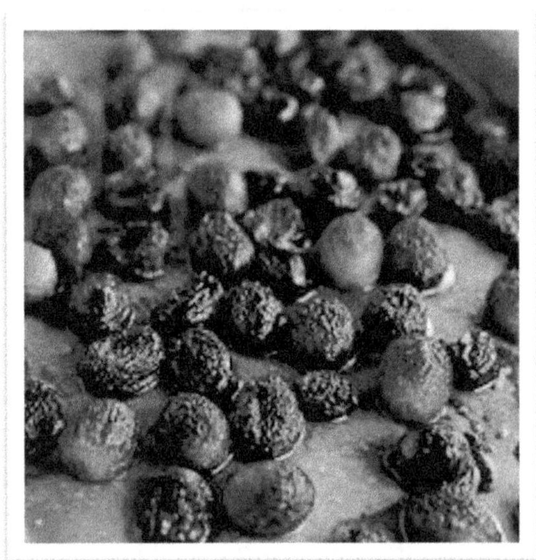

Calories: 12 kcal| Total time: 25 minutes| Servings: 12|Difficulty: Easy

Ingredients

- Balsamic vinegar, 1/3 cup

- Olive oil, 3 tablespoons

- Brown sugar, 1 teaspoon

- Fresh thyme, 1 teaspoon

- Black pepper, 1/2 teaspoon

- Fresh seedless grapes, 1/2 lb.

- Mascarpone, 6 oz

- French bread, 12 slices

Instructions

1. Preheat oven to 400°. Toss grapes, thyme, and olive oil in a lined baking sheet. Season with pepper. Roast for 15 minutes and stirring occasionally. Bake till grapes are softened.

2. Brush baguette slices with remaining olive oil. Place on the baking sheet bake for

   8 minutes.

3. Reduce the vinegar overheat till it thickens and reduces to 2 Tablespoon. Stir brown sugar and add black pepper.

4. Spread mascarpone cheese onto the toast. Place the grapes on top and drizzle with balsamic vinegar.

5. Serve.

4. Kidney friendly Chia seed pudding

Calories: 100 kcal| Total time: 20 minutes| Servings: 4|Difficulty: Easy

Ingredients

- 1/2 cup, Chia Seeds

- 1 teaspoon, Vanilla Extract

- 1/4 cup Maple Syrup

- 1/4 teaspoon, Cinnamon

- 1 1/2 cup, Rice Milk

Instructions

1. In a bowl, combine all ingredients.

2. Stir chia mixture making sure seeds do not stick to sides of the container.

3. Cover and put in the refrigerator.

4. Serve.

5. Kidney friend Fruit Crunch

Calories: 217 kcal| Total time: 20 minutes| Servings: 4|Difficulty: Easy

Ingredients

- Tart apples, 4 large, cored and sliced.

- sugar, ¾ cup

- All-purpose flour, ½ cups, sifted.

- Margarine, ⅓ cup, softened.

- Rolled oats, ¾ cup

- nutmeg, ¾ teaspoon

Instructions

1. Preheat oven to 375°F.

2. Place apples in a greased pan.

3. Combine all ingredients in a bowl, spread over fruit.

4. Now bake for 30-35 minutes.

5. Serve.

6. Blueberry Baked Bread

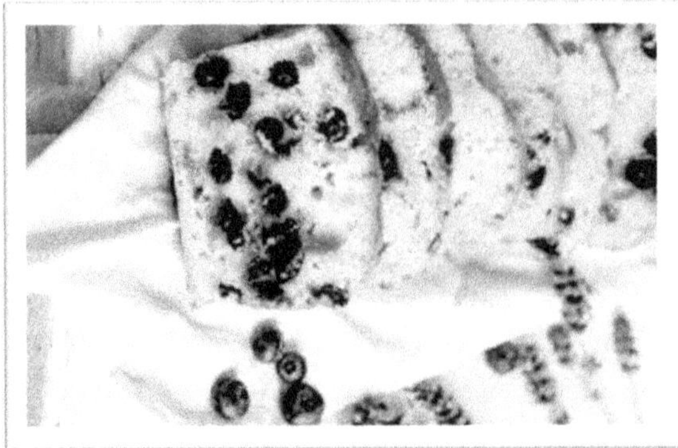

Calories: 176 kcal| Total time: 20 minutes| Servings: 6|Difficulty: Easy

Ingredients

- Blueberries, 1 quart, fresh or frozen
- Water, ¼ cup
- Lemon juice, 1 teaspoon
- Sugar, ½ cup
- Nutmeg, 1 pinch
- Cinnamon, 1 pinch
- Margarine, 1 tablespoon
- Bread, 3 slices, buttered, cut into pieces

Directions

1. Heat the oven to about 425ºF.
2. Combine all ingredients except bread in a pan. Bring to boil.
3. Pour mixture into a baking pan, top with bread pieces.
4. Bake until brown.
5. Serve.

7. Smart and Sweet Popcorn

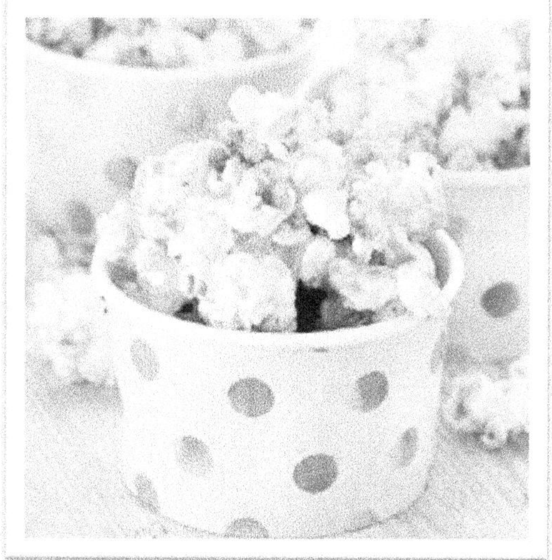

Calories: 176 kcal| Total time: 20 minutes| Servings: 6|Difficulty: Easy

Ingredients

- Microwave popcorn, 12 cups
- Cooking spray
- Cumin, 1½ teaspoons
- Garlic powder, 1 teaspoon
- Onion powder, 1 teaspoon
- Worcestershire sauce, 1½ teaspoons
- Brown sugar, 1/2 teaspoon
- Paprika, 1/2 teaspoon
- Cayenne pepper, 1 teaspoon

Directions

1. Preheat the oven to 250 °C.

2. Place popcorn in a bowl. Lightly spray them with the cooking spray.

3. Combine all spices and sprinkle over popcorn.

4. Mix Worcestershire sauce with brown sugar until sugar dissolves and sprinkle it over popcorn.

5. Spread the popcorn in a baking pan.

6. Bake for almost 10 minutes.

7. Serve hot.

---

8 Kidney friendly Very Veggie Dip

Calories: 50 kcal| Total time: 10 minutes| Servings: 10|Difficulty: Easy

Ingredients

- Light cream cheese, 8-ounce package, softened
- Fat-free sour cream, 1/4 cup
- Garlic powder, 1/4 teaspoon
- Grated parmesan cheese, 2 tablespoons

- Chives, finely chopped, 1/4 cup

- Red peppers, diced, 1/4 cup

- Worcestershire sauce, 1 tablespoon

Instructions

1. Combine all ingredients and mix.

2. Then cover and place in the refrigerator.

3. Serve with your favorite vegetables.

9. Roasted Chickpeas

Calories: 50 kcal| Total time: 20 minutes| Servings: 10|Difficulty: Easy

Ingredients

- Chickpeas, canned, 15 ounces

- Salt, 1/8 teaspoon

- Garlic powder, 1 teaspoon

- Olive oil, 2 teaspoons

Instructions

1. Preheat the oven to 375° F. Drain, rinse, and pat dry chickpeas.

2. Place chickpeas on a baking sheet and bake for 30 to 35 minutes. Shake the pan after every 1o minutes.

3. In a bowl, combine salt garlic powder. Remove chickpeas when done and sprinkle with olive oil.

4. Serve.

10. Egg sausage sandwiches

Calories: 250 kcal| Total time: 20 minutes| Servings: 2|Difficulty: Easy

Ingredients

- Egg substitute, 1/4 cup

- English muffin, 1

- Turkey sausage patty, 1

- Shredded cheddar cheese, 1 tablespoon

Preparation

1. Pour egg product into a skillet and cook on low to medium heat. Cook the egg.

2. Toast English muffin.

3. Place turkey sausage on a plate and cook in the microwave for about 1 minute.

4. Place cooked egg on the English muffin. Top with a sausage patty.

5. Cut into half, spread cheese, and serve.

---

11. Classic blueberry scones

Calories: 153 kcal| Total time: 40 minutes| Servings: 12|Difficulty: Easy

Ingredients

- Almond Flour, 2 cups

- Swerve sweetener, 1/3 cup

- Coconut flour, 1/4 cup

- Baking powder, 1 tablespoon

- Salt, 1/4 teaspoon

- Large eggs, 2

- Whipping cream, 1/4 cup

- Vanilla extract, 1/2 teaspoon

- Fresh blueberries, 3/4 cup

Instructions

1. To 325F, preheat the oven and line with parchment a big baking sheet or silicone lining.

2. Whisk the sweetener, almond flour, baking powder, coconut flour, and salt together in a big pot.

3. Add the eggs, mixing the cream and the vanilla, then blend until the dough starts to fit. Attach the blueberries, then function through the dough carefully. Assemble the dough and transfer it to the baking dish. Pat into a 10 x 8-inch rectangle.

4. Using a big, sharp knife to cut in 6 squares. Then diagonally split one of those squares into 2 triangles. Pick the scones softly and scatter them across the oven. Bake for 20-25 mins, till brown (golden) and firm it should be. Remove and allow to cool.

5. Serve

Graham crackers Calories: 156 kcal| Total time: 20 minutes| Servings: 10|Difficulty: Easy

Ingredients

- Almond flour 2 cups

- Swerve brown 1/3 cup

- Cinnamon es2 teaspoon

- Baking powder 1 teaspoon

- Pinch salt

- Large egg 1

- Butter melted 2 tablespoons

- Vanilla extract 1 teaspoon

Instructions

1. The oven preheated to 300 F.

2. Whisk the coconut flour, sweetener, spice, baking powder & salt together in a big dish.

3. Add the sugar, softened butter, black treacle & vanilla extract before the dough is combined.

4. Place the dough onto a wide sheet of bakery release paper or filler it with silicone, then pat it into a harsh rectangle. Cover it with such a single sheet of paper. Roll the dough as thinly if possible, To a thickness of around 1/8-1/4 inches.

5. Take off the top parchment & use the knife or even a pizza.

6. Cutter to grade approximately 2 × 2 inches into squares. Place the whole parchment on a

cookie sheet.

7. Bake for 20-30 mins, till it becomes brown & strong. Remove crackers, let them cool for 30 Mins, then break down together with score points. Go to a warm oven. Let mix it for the other 30 mins, then allow It to cool fully (they crisp up while they cool).

8. Strawberry cheesecake popsicles – low carb and gluten-free

Calories: 122 kcal| Total time: 4 hrs. 15 min| Servings: 12|Difficulty: hard

Ingredients

- Softened cream cheese, 8 oz

- Cream, 1 cup

- Powdered Swerve sweetener 1/3 cup

- Stevia extract, 1/4 teaspoon

- Lemon juice, 1 tablespoon

- Lemon zest, 2 teaspoons

- Chopped fresh strawberries, 2 cups

Instructions

1. Place and heat your "cream-cheese" In the mixing bowl till smooth.

2. Add milk powder swerve, lime Juice, stevia extract & lemon zest. Mixed phase till well.

3. Attach 1 1/2 cups of raspberries & finish processing until completely smooth. Delete Sliced leftover raspberries.

4. Pour the mixture into molds of popsicle & push Sticks of popsicle around two/three of the way in each.

5. Freeze it for 4 hrs. Run for 20-30 seconds under warm water to unmold, after which turn stick nicely to release.

14. Bagel cucumber bites

Calories: 93 kcal| Total time: 25 minutes| Servings: 8|Difficulty: Medium

Ingredients

- Poppy seeds, 1 teaspoon

- Sesame seeds, 1 teaspoon

- Dried minced garlic, 1/2 teaspoon

- Dried minced onion, 1/2 teaspoon

- Crushed caraway seeds, 1/4 teaspoon

- Coarse salt, 1/4 teaspoon

- Medium cucumber, 1

- Cream cheese, 4 ounces

- Butter softened, 2 tablespoons

- Greek yogurt, 2 tablespoons

- Garlic powder, 1/2 teaspoon

- Salt, 1/4 teaspoon

Instructions

1. Whisk all of the ingredients with Each other in a bowl. Place On aside.

2. Use a fine knife to Cut off the cucumber. Cross-slice that cucumber into 1/4 "thick Pieces & placed them on the platter.

3. Hit the cream cheese, butter, milk, garlic powder & salt in a med bowl till they are well mixed and smooth.

4. Attach a star-shaped tip to the piping bag & Fill the bag with a combination of cream cheese. Decoratively pouring the Cucumber slices on top.

5. Sprinkle with all bagel seasoning on every slice and serve

15. Homemade renal friendly sausage

Calories: 93 kcal| Total time: 25 minutes| Servings: 8|Difficulty: Medium

Ingredients

- Onion, 1⁄2 cup, finely chopped
- Olive oil, 2 tablespoons
- Dried sage, 2 teaspoons
- Fresh ground 1 teaspoon, black pepper
- Sugar, 1 tablespoon
- Red pepper flakes, 1⁄8 teaspoon
- Ground cloves, 1 pinch
- Fresh thyme, 1 teaspoon, finely chopped.
- Egg yolk, 1 large
- Lean pork, 2 lbs. ground

Directions

1. Cook onion in olive oil on moderately low heat till soft and brown. Cool them for 10 minutes.
2. Combine sage, pepper, sugar, thyme, and cloves in a bowl.
3. Place egg yolk, reserved onion and pork in a large bowl and add mixed spices.
4. Make 16 patties.
5. Pan fry them in a large skillet for 5 minutes on both sides.
6. Serve.

16. Kidney friendly fruit dip

Calories: 123 kcal| Total time: 20 minutes| Servings: 10|Difficulty: Easy

Ingredients

- Sour Cream, 1 Cup, (Low phosphorous dip)
- Brown Sugar, 2 Tablespoon
- Vanilla Extract, 1/2 Teaspoon

Instructions

1. Mix brown sugar, sour cream, and vanilla extract.

2. Let it stand in a refrigerator for the flavors to combine (at least 1 hr. or 2 hr. or better overnight).

3. Cut all fruits such as bananas, grapes, apples, melon, oranges, strawberries, peaches, pears, or watermelon into chunks or as desired.

4. To prevent discoloration, Dip apples, bananas in some lemon juice.

5. Place the fruit at the edge of serving dish.

6. Place the dip in dish in enter of tray.

17. Heavenly Deviled Eggs

Calories: 98 kcal| Total time: 10 minutes| Servings: 4|Difficulty: Easy

Ingredients

- Eggs, hard boiled, shells removed, 4 large

- Light mayonnaise, 2 tablespoons

- Dry mustard, ½ teaspoon

- Cider vinegar, ½ teaspoon

- Onion, finely chopped, 1 tablespoon

- Ground black pepper, ¼ teaspoon

- Dash of paprika, optional garnish

Directions

1. Cut the eggs into half, lengthwise. Now carefully remove the yolks and place them in small bowl. Transfer egg white in a plate.

2. Mix yolks with the help of fork and add vinegar, onion, dry mustard, and black pepper.

3. Now refill the egg white with the yolk mixture, piling slightly.

4. Finally sprinkle the deviled eggs with some paprika.

5. Serve.

---

18. Sweet & Nutty Protein Bars

Calories: 283 kcal| Total time: 30 minutes| Servings: 8|Difficulty: Easy

Ingredients

- Rolled oats, toasted, 2½ cups

- Almonds, ½ cup

- Flaxseeds, ½ cup

- Peanut butter, ½ cup

- Dried cherries, 1 cup, blueberries or craisins®

- Honey, ½ cup

Instructions

1. Toast the oats by placing rolled oats on a baking sheet in a 350° F oven for 10 minutes or until golden brown.

2. Mix all ingredients together until well-mixed.

3. Press the protein mix down into a lightly greased 9" x 9" pan. Wrap and refrigerate for at least one hour or overnight.

4. Cut protein bars into desired squares then serve.

---

19. Crispy Cauliflower Phyllo Cups

Calories: 283 kcal| Total time: 30 minutes| Servings: 8|Difficulty: Easy

Ingredients

- Beaten, lightly scrambled, 3 eggs

- Swiss cheese, ½ cup, shredded

- Cheddar cheese, ½ cup, shredded

- Butter, 2 tablespoons

- Natural and uncured, 4 slices bacon, diced

- Cauliflower, diced, cooked, 1½ cups

- Onions, finely diced, ¼ cup

- Jalapeños, diced, 2 tablespoons

- Red pepper flakes, ½ teaspoon

- Parsley, 1 tablespoon

- Ground black pepper, ½ teaspoon

- Phyllo dough, 3 sheets

- Parsley, black pepper, optional garnish

Instructions

1. Preheat the oven to 375° F.

2. In a large pan, scramble the eggs, then remove them and set aside.

3. In same pan, melt the butter and sauté bacon till cooked. Add onions, jalapeños, cauliflower, and red pepper, sauté till the onions become translucent. Now season with ground black pepper parsley.

4. Then remove from the heat and add scrambled eggs and two cheeses.

5. Now layer three phyllo sheets and cut the sheets in 24 squares, press lightly on mini muffin tin pan.

6. Now fill each cup with same amounts of mix, bake on bottom shelf of oven for almost 12 to 15 minutes, or till slightly golden. Turn off the oven and let them rest for almost 2–3 minutes.

7. Serve.

20. Kidney friendly Orange and Cinnamon Biscotti

Calories: 273 kcal| Total time: 1 hr. 8 minutes| Servings: 8|Difficulty: Easy

Ingredients

- Sugar, 1 cup

- Unsalted butter, room temperature, ½ cup

- Eggs, 2 large

- Grated orange peel, 2 teaspoons

- Vanilla extract, 1 teaspoon

- All-purpose flour, 2 cups

- Cream of tartar, 1 teaspoon

- Baking soda, ½ teaspoon

- Ground cinnamon, 1 teaspoon

- Salt, ¼ teaspoon

Instructions

1. Preheat the oven to 325° F.

2. Spray two baking sheets using nonstick cooking spray.

3. Beat the sugar & unsalted butter in large bowl till well blended.

4. Now add eggs 1 at a time, beat well after each.

5. Add in orange peel & vanilla.

6. Now mix flour, baking soda, cream of tartar, cinnamon, and salt.

7. Then add dry ingredients to the butter mixture and then mix until completely incorporated.

8. Now divide the dough in half. Put each half in a sheet. With floured hands, make each half to log shape which is three inches wide by 3 quarters of the inch high. Then bake till the dough logs become firm to touch, around 35 minutes.

9. Now remove the dough logs from the oven and cool them for 10 minutes.

10. Then transfer the logs to a surface. By using knife, cut ½-inch-thick slices in diagonal. Arrange the cut side down on the baking sheets.

11. Now bake till the bottoms turns golden, around 12 minutes.

12. Flip biscotti over; then bake till bottoms are golden, around 12 minutes longer.

13. Take out from the wire rack, cool

14. Serve.

21. Sweat cornbread muffins

Calories: 216 kcal| Total time: 30 minutes| Servings: 12|Difficulty: Easy

Ingredients

- Cornmeal, 1 cup

- Flour, 1 cup

- Baking soda, 1 ½ teaspoons

- Lemon juice, 3 tablespoons

- Egg, beaten, 1

- Milk, 1 cup

- Unsalted butter, melted, ½ stick

- Vanilla extract, 1 tablespoon

- Honey Butter:

- Honey, 2 tablespoons

- Unsalted butter, softened, 1 stick

- Orange zest, ½ teaspoon

- Black pepper, ¼ teaspoon

- Orange extract, ½ teaspoon

Instructions

1. Preheat the oven to 400° F.

2. In a bowl, beat milk, butter & egg together till mixed well.

3. In another bowl, mix cornmeal, baking soda & flour then mix both dry and liquid ingredients till smooth. Be sure do not overbeat.

4. Now line muffin tins with a muffin liner, then ill each cup with ¾ full & bake for around 15–20 minutes, place in the middle rack.

5. In a separate bowl, mix the honey butter ingredients till properly blended and spread on the top of the cornbread muffins

6. Serve the honey butter on side if you like.

22. kidney friendly Mama Chipotle Wings

Calories: 216 kcal| Total time: 30 minutes| Servings: 12|Difficulty: Easy

Ingredients

- Fresh big chicken wings, 1 pound, cut in pieces, 20 individual pieces

- Some oil, greasing baking tray's sheet

- Diced chipotle peppers, 1½ tablespoons, in adobo sauce

- Honey, ¼ cup

- Unsalted butter, ¼ cup, slightly melted

- Black pepper, 1 teaspoon

- Chopped chives, 1 tablespoon

Instructions

1. Preheat the oven to 400° F.

2. Put the precut wings over a large, greased baking sheet tray (nonstick).

3. Bake for around 18–20 minutes, keep on turning halfway during the cooking time, until crispy from the outside & reaching an interior temperature of 165° F in an instantaneous-read thermometer.

4. Transfer the remaining ingredients in a large bowl & combine with the help of rubber spatula, till well mixed.

5. Finally, remove wings from oven & toss till evenly coated.

6. Transfer in a large platter.

7. Serve and Enjoy.

23. Barbecue Turkey Wings

Calories: 293 kcal| Total time: 1 hr. 30 minutes| Servings: 12|Difficulty: Easy

Ingredients

- Turkey wings, 7 whole

- Barbecue spice rub (mix all the ingredients together):

- Dark brown sugar, 1 cup packed

- Black pepper, 1 teaspoon

- Red pepper flakes, 1 teaspoon

- Smoked paprika, 1 teaspoon

- Granulated garlic, 2 teaspoons

- Dehydrated onion flakes, 2 teaspoons

- Dark chili powder, 2 teaspoons

- Favorite low sodium barbecue sauce (two tablespoons/ wing), 14 tablespoons.

Instructions

1. Preheat the oven to 375° F.

2. Start patting the wings dry & pierce them with fork from both sides.

3. Now rub the wings generously with spice rub, save 1 tablespoon.

4. Now place the wings on baking tray & bake wrapped in foil for around 30 minutes. Then remove wings from the oven & discard foil, then flip over & cook for 30 minutes more. Now sprinkle the rest of the seasoning on wings & flip back over.

5. Lastly, turn off the oven & let sit in oven for around 15 minutes,

6. Then serve with your favorite low sodium barbecue sauce.

7. Enjoy your time.

24. Dried Cranberry Fruit Bars

Calories: 130 kcal| Total time: 40 minutes| Servings: 24|Difficulty: Easy

Ingredients

Crust:

- All-purpose flour, 1 ½ cups

- Sugar, 1 1/3 cups

- Unsalted butter (1 1/2 sticks), ¾ cup

Topping:

- All-purpose flour, ½ cup

- Baking powder, 1 teaspoon

- Dried cranberries, 1 cup

- Sugar, ¾ cup

- Eggs, 4 large

- Vanilla extract, 1 teaspoon

- For dusting, powdered sugar (optional)

Instructions

1. Preheat the oven to 350° F.

2. In a medium-size bowl, mix sugar & flour together; now cut the unsalted butter till the mixture clings together. Now pat it on an ungreased 9" by 13" baking pan. Then bake for around 10 minutes till becomes lightly brown.

3. In a small bowl, prepare topping, sift the flour & baking powder together. Now toss in some dried cranberries & set aside.

4. In a medium-sized bowl, combine sugar, eggs & vanilla. Then add flour mixture. Then pour it into baked crust. Now cake for about 20 to 25 minutes.

5. After this, cut 24 bars when it is still warm & dust with some powdered sugar.

Serve and Enjoy

25. Kidney friendly Chocolate popcorn bars

Calories: 130 kcal| Total time: 40 minutes| Servings: 24|Difficulty: Easy

Ingredients

- Organic popcorn kernels, 1/2 cup

- Allergy-friendly chocolate chips, 6 ounces, like mini chips (1 cup)

- Sea salt, 1/2 teaspoon

Instructions

1. Pop the popcorn kernels by following the manufacturer's instructions. The best option is to pop in electric air popper. 12 cups of the popped popcorns will be prepared by doing this. Now place them in a big bowl & set aside.

2. Now fill a saucepan with water & bring to boil. Then put chocolate in a separate bowl; bowl of chocolate must not be in straight contact with water. After placing the bowl on saucepan, lesser the heat so that the water starts to gently simmer. Melt chocolate and keep on stirring occasionally.

3. Now remove melted chocolate from the heat. Then wipe bottom of bowl and dry any condensation. Instantly pour it over the popcorn then stir to coat thoroughly as possible. Do wear disposable vinyl gloves and toss with your hands.

4. Now spread it evenly onto the baking sheet that must line with the parchment paper. Now sprinkle with sea salt. Lastly, let sit at around room temperature till the chocolate hardens & sets, for about an hour.

5. You can keep this for up to three days in a sealed container.

Conclusion

A kidney-friendly or renal diet is a healthy diet that serves to protect kidneys against damage. For chronic kidney disease, there is currently no proven treatment, but there are habits and activities which can reduce the progression of renal failure, including lifestyle behaviors. For those who suffer from diabetes, heart disease, high blood pressure, or have a history of kidney failure, they are already at the risk for kidney disease. You must now know that correct levels of nutrients, calories, vitamins, and minerals are very essential. This book has provided a range of kidney-friendly recipes that will help you maintain sodium, phosphorus, and potassium levels in the body. To cut the salt in your diet is necessary, as the body accumulates additional sodium & fluids. It can exacerbate various conditions of heart and lungs such as swelling of knees, elevated blood pressure, fluid buildup, and shortness of breath. The amounts of not more than 1,000 milligrams (mg) of phosphorus mineral per day in late-stage CKD that can be achieved by having chosen foods with low phosphorus levels such as, consuming additional new vegetables and fruit, selecting cereals including corn and rice, light-colored drinking sodas, trying to cut back on beef, seafood, and poultry and restriction of dairy foods. One must make more adjustments to the diet if CKD becomes worse. It may mean cutting back on high-protein foods, particularly animal protein. It involves items such as beef, fish, including dairy. Based on these recommendations this book has provided recipes that include many options for breakfast, lunch, and dinner. You must also have learned some easy to make and delicious recipes for snacks, salads, desserts, and beverages. We hope that by trying these recipes you must have put a lot of fun to your kitchen and dining table. We hope that this recipe book must have brought a great change in your daily eating habits and a good change in your body. Keep on trying these recipes in your daily routine and have a good and healthy life ahead. Because healthy food will keep you away from the complications of renal issues.

Your feedback is very valuable to us. It gives us support in bringing healthy and delicious recipes for you and your family. Do not forget to provide your honest review. We highly appreciate it.

Thank you.

www.ingramcontent.com/pod-product-compliance
Lightning Source LLC
Chambersburg PA
CBHW081610250726
48657CB00009B/2531